Spasticity Rehabilitation

Spasticity Rehabilitation

Edited by

Geoffrey Sheean MBBS FRACP

Consultant in Clinical Neurophysiology
The National Hospital for Neurology and Neurosurgery
Queen Square, London, UK

Foreword by

Michael P. Barnes MD FRCP

Professor of Neurological Rehabilitation
Hunters Moor Regional Rehabilitation Centre
University of Newcastle
Newcastle, UK

FIRST EDITION

 CHURCHILL COMMUNICATIONS
EUROPE LTD

CHURCHILL COMMUNICATIONS EUROPE LIMITED
A Division of Quadrant Healthcom Inc.

© Churchill Communications Europe Ltd 1998

First published 1998

ISBN 1 902446 00 3

British Library Cataloguing in Publication Data
A catalogue record for this book is available from the British Library.

Library of Congress Cataloguing in Publication Data
A catalog record for this book is available from the Library of Congress.

Note
Medical knowledge is constantly changing. As new information becomes available, changes in treatment, procedures, equipment and the use of drugs become necessary. The editor, authors, sponsor and the publishers have, as far as it is possible, taken care to ensure that the information given in this text is accurate and up to date. However, readers are strongly advised to confirm that the information, especially with regard to drug usage, complies with latest legislation and standards of practice.

Neither the publishers nor the authors will be liable for any loss or damage of any nature occasioned to or suffered by any person acting or refraining from acting as a result of reliance on the material contained in this publication.

Typeset by Saxon Graphics Ltd, Derby, UK
Printed in Great Britain at Biddles Ltd, Guildford

Contents

Foreword

It is a pleasure to write a Foreword for this important book. Spasticity is a major rehabilitation problem. Active and appropriate treatment can lead to a significant improvement in the quality of life both for the disabled person and carer. Yet, despite recent advances, it is often poorly treated and mismanaged and this can lead to unnecessary functional problems, pain and increasing and unnecessary disability and handicap. This book seeks to correct a significant gap in the general knowledge of clinicians. It is a practical book, full of sensible, straightforward guidance on the therapy and the medical and surgical management of spasticity. However, the authors have not forgotten the basic principles and cover the pathophysiology and importance of clinical measurement. This is an excellent book and one which I am sure you will enjoy reading and learn much from.

MPB
January 1998

Contributors

Susan Edwards
Clinical Specialist, Physiotherapy, The National Hospital for
Neurology and Neurosurgery, Queen Square, London, UK

Richard Greenwood MD
Consultant in Clinical Neurology to the National Hospital for
Neurology and Neurosurgery, Queen Square, The Homerton
Hospital, and The Homerton Regional Neurological
Rehabilitation Unit, London, UK

Davina Richardson
Research Physiotherapist, The National Hospital for Neurology
and Neurosurgery, Queen Square, London, UK

Geoffrey L. Sheean MBBS FRACP
Consultant in Clinical Neurophysiology, The National Hospital for
Neurology and Neurosurgery, Queen Square, London, UK

Alan J. Thompson MD
Professor of Clinical Neurology and Neurorehabilitation and
Director of Neurorehabilitation and Therapy Services, The
National Hospital for Neurology and Neurosurgery, Queen Square,
London, UK

David J. Werring BSc MRCP(UK)
Neurology Research Fellow, The National Hospital for Neurology
and Neurosurgery, Queen Square, Specialist Registrar in
Neurology, The Whittington Hospital, London, UK

ticity may also reduce the other UMN hypertonias seen at rest that result from peripheral stimulation, but are unlikely to affect those generated centrally, comprising the spastic dystonias and spastic synergies, which dominate the picture, at least in functional settings, after cerebral damage. It is logical therefore to expect baclofen, for example, to be more effective in relieving the hypertonia of spinal rather than cerebral UMN syndromes,[23] whilst factors other than the nature of the tone increase will limit the effectiveness of treatments such as BTX.

The treatments available for spasticity and the other forms of muscle hypertonias seen in the UMN syndrome are increasing in number. Intramuscular injections of BTX or the prescription of oral or intrathecal baclofen offer opportunities for clinical activity which may or may not always result in useful gains. This book intends to practically illustrate how these treatments should or should not be deployed and why they may or may not be successful in an individual patient. It is the product of multidisciplinary clinical effort. We hope it illustrates the lessons we have learned and suggests ways in which integrated treatment of aspects of the UMN syndrome is more likely to result in benefit than treatment of spasticity alone.

REFERENCES

1. Thilmann AF 1993 Spasticity: history, definitions, and usage of the term. In: Thilmann AF, Burke DJ, Rymer WZ (eds) Spasticity: mechanisms and management. Springer-Verlag, Berlin, pp 1–5
2. Burridge JH, Taylor PN, Hagan SA, Wood DE, Swain ID 1997 The effects of common peroneal stimulation on the effort and speed of walking: a randomised controlled trial with chronic hemiplegic patients. Clin Rehabil 11: 201–210
3. Thilmann AF, Fellows SJ, Garms E 1991 The mechanisms of spastic muscle hypertonus. Variation in reflex gain over the time course of spasticity. Brain 114: 233–244
4. Burke D, Gillies JD, Lance JW 1970 The quadriceps stretch reflex in human spasticity. J Neurol Neurosurg Psychiatry 33: 216–223
5. Hagbarth KE, Wallin G, Lofstedt L 1973 Muscle spindle responses to stretch in normal and spastic subjects. Scand J Rehab Med 5: 156–159
6. Brown P 1994 Pathophysiology of spasticity. J Neurol Neurosurg Psychiatry 57: 773–777
7. Lance JW 1994 What is spasticity? Lancet I: 606
8. Powers RK, Marder-Meyer J, Rymer WZ 1988 Quantitative relations between hypertonia and stretch reflex threshold in spastic hemiparesis. Ann Neurol 23: 115–124
9. Powers RK, Campbell DL, Rymer WZ 1989 Stretch reflex dynamics in spastic elbow flexor muscles. Ann Neurol 25: 32–42
10. Gottlieb GL, Myklebust BM 1993 Hyper-reflexis and disordered voluntary movement. In: Thilmann AF, Burke DJ, Rymer WZ (eds) Spasticity: mechanisms and management. Springer-Verlag, Berlin, pp 155–156

11. Dietz V, Quinten J, Berger W 1981 Electrophysiological studies of gait in spasticity rigidity. Evidence that altered mechanical properties of muscle contribute to hypertonia. Brain 104: 431–449
12. Given JD, Dewald JPA, Rymer WZ 1995 Joint dependent passive stiffness in paretic and contralateral limbs of spastic patients with hemiparetic stroke. J Neurol Neurosurg Psychiatry 59: 271–279
13. Brunnstrom S 1970 Movement therapy in hemiplegia. Harper & Row, New York.
14. Denny-Brown D 1966 The cerebral control of movement. Liverpool University Press, Liverpool, pp 170–184
15. Benecke R, Conrad B, Meinck HM, Hohne J 1983 Electromyographic analysis of bicycling on an ergometer for evaluation of spasticity of lower limbs in man. In: Desmedt JE (ed) Motor control mechanisms in health and disease. Raven Press, New York, pp 1035–1046
16. Corcos DM, Gottleib GL, Penn RD, Myklebust B, Agarwal GC 1986 Movement deficits caused by hyperexcitable stretch reflexes in spastic humans. Brain 109: 1043–1058
17. Landau WM 1974 Spasticity: the fable of a neurological demon and the emperor's new therapy. Ann Neurol 31: 217–219
18. Young RR, Delwaide PJ 1981 Drug therapy: spasticity (first of two parts). N Engl J Med 304: 28–33
19. Lance JW 1980 Pathophysiology of spasticity and clinical experience with baclofen. In: Feldman RG, Young RR, Koella WP (eds) Spasticity: disordered motor control. Year Book Medical Publishers, Chicago, pp 185–203
20. Twitchell TE 1951 The restoration of motor function following hemiplegia in man. Brain 74: 443–480
21. Walshe FMR 1923 On certain tonic or postural reflexes in hemiplegia, with special reference to the so-called 'associated movements'. Brain 46: 1–37
22. Dimitrijevic MR, Faganel J, Sherwood AM, McKay WB 1981 Activation of paralysed leg flexors and extensors during gait in patients after stroke. Scand J Rehab Med 13: 109–115
23. Young RR, Delwaide PJ 1981 Drug therapy: spasticity (second of two parts). N Engl J Med 304: 96–99

2. Clinical features of spasticity and the upper motor neurone syndrome

Geoffrey L. Sheean

INTRODUCTION

The term spasticity (derived from the Greek *spastikos* meaning to tug or draw) may conjure up in many clinicians' minds several quite different clinical images. This is despite spasticity having been given a fairly strict and narrow, physiologically based definition some years ago by Lance:[1]

> *'Spasticity is a motor disorder characterized by a velocity-dependent increase in tonic stretch reflexes ('muscle tone') with exaggerated tendon jerks, resulting from hyperexcitability of the stretch reflex, as one component of the upper motor neurone syndrome.'*

The first chapter introduced the concept of the upper motor neurone (UMN) syndrome, emphasising that spasticity is only one of its components. This chapter will discuss its clinical features in more detail. The pathophysiology of spasticity and the UMN syndrome and their overall clinical impact will be discussed in subsequent chapters.

DEFINITION OF THE UMN SYNDROME

The UMN syndrome is a somewhat vague but useful concept because its numerous clinical features have not yet been fully assigned to the many candidate descending motor pathways. UMNs are those in any long descending tract that control or influence movement and muscle tone, having a more or less direct influence upon the excitability of the lower motor neurone (Table 3.1). The UMN syndrome is caused by lesions affecting some or all of these pathways.

prone to developing decreased compliance of these tissues, which may dominate the picture. Biomechanical hypertonia is not velocity dependent and may restrict movement even at slow angular velocities. Furthermore, this form of hypertonia will not respond to anti-spastic agents and is best treated by physiotherapy. It can be difficult to distinguish clinically between spasticity and reduced muscle compliance. There is the velocity dependence of spasticity and a distinctive stiff, elastic 'feel' to the hypertonia of reduced muscle compliance. In practice there is often a mixture of each, and EMG is particularly useful in determining their relative contributions to the hypertonia, without having to resort to anaesthesia or nerve blocks.

These changes in the visco-elastic properties of the muscle and adjacent tissues may increase tone but still allow a full passive range of joint movement. Muscle contractures may represent the extreme form of these biomechanical changes, in which there is fixed shortening of the muscle and a reduced passive range of movement. In some cases with contracture and a reduced range of movement there is surprisingly normal tone, indicating that reduced compliance and contractures are related but separate phenomena. Spasticity is not the sole cause of contractures.[2] Contractures arise from prolonged maintenance of a muscle in a shortened position and may owe as much or more to poor positioning of a weakened limb as to spasticity or flexor spasms.

Hyperactive tendon reflexes and clonus

Tendon hyperreflexia so frequently accompanies spasticity that the two are often, erroneously, considered synonymous. Tendon hyperreflexia is also commonly taken as evidence that hypertonia is spasticity rather than rigidity. Tendon hyperreflexia and spasticity may be clinically dissociated, however, and their pathophysiological mechanisms are not exactly the same. Hyperactive reflexes may also be seen in pathological conditions other than the UMN syndrome (e.g. hyperthyroidism) and in some nervous but healthy individuals. In these states, as well as in the UMN syndrome, there may be radiation of the reflexes. For example, tapping the Achilles tendon of one leg may cause a brisk jerk-like contraction of the quadriceps and adductors of the same leg and even the adductors of the opposite leg (a 'crossed-adductor reflex').

Clonus is a variant of tendon hyperreflexia, most often seen at the ankle. A sharp passive dorsiflexion of the ankle with the limb positioned correctly may elicit a rhythmic contraction of the plantarflexors (clonus) that may continue for as long as the dorsiflexion pressure is maintained (sustained clonus). Unsustained clonus is often considered non-pathological but can be seen in the UMN syndrome, just as both may occur in the other pathological and 'physiological' states that can cause hyperactive tendon jerks. Whether clonus is present and then sustained or unsustained depends greatly on technique.[3] Clonus is always accompanied by hyperactive tendon jerks, but not necessarily vice versa; its presence provides no more diagnostic information than that obtained from the tendon reflexes. Hyperactive tendon jerks are a physical sign with no functional clinical significance but clonus at the ankle can interfere with standing and walking.

Flexor spasms

Strong spasms of the hip, knee and ankle flexors can occur apparently spontaneously or in response to cutaneous stimulation. Such stimulation need not be noxious; even the weight of bedclothes on the legs can evoke spasms. In addition to flexion, there may be adduction and internal rotation of the thigh. Flexor spasms are more frequently seen with spinal cord lesions than with cerebral lesions, for reasons outlined in Chapter 3. They may be quite painful and so severe as to produce a permanent state of flexion (paraplegia-in-flexion). Common aggravating factors are bedsores and bladder infections. Distension of the bowel or bladder can also produce flexor spasms and severe spasms may be accompanied by reflex emptying of these structures ('mass reflex'). Non-specific stimulation such as coughing or sneezing can also evoke spasms. Aside from causing pain, flexor spasms create difficulty with standing and walking, dressing, positioning (e.g. seating) and general nursing care. They may also place the patient at risk of contracture.

Extensor spasms

Muscle spasms producing extension of the hip and knee, with plantarflexion and possibly inversion of the ankle, may also occur in the UMN syndrome. Extensor spasms, as with flexor spasms, can be painful, interfere with nursing care and dressing and be disabling, interfering with standing and walking. Extensor spasms are more likely with incomplete spinal lesions (paraplegia-in-extension) and cerebral lesions, than with complete spinal cord lesions. However, various stimuli that evoke flexor spasms can convert the posture from extension to flexion.[4] Similarly, stimulation of the skin overlying extensor muscles[5] and iliopsoas stretch are potent stimuli to extensor spasms.

Extensor spasms occur in other forms. The upright hemiplegic posture includes extension of the leg and can be viewed as a form of extensor spasm. A unilateral flexor withdrawal reflex is often accompanied by extension of the opposite leg. The positive supporting reaction is also a type of extensor spasm. Placing pressure on the ball of the foot to stand or walk produces strong extension of the leg, turning it into a rigid pillar. In milder forms this may provide a supporting 'splint' to help the patient stand by performing crutch duties but, when severe, can make it impossible to stand or walk and can even propel the patient backwards. The reflex may make it impossible for the heel to touch the floor or for the patient to move forward over the leg when walking without requiring marked hip flexion to compensate. Such a posture may lead in time to shortening of the hip flexors as well as the knee extensors and ankle plantarflexors. This reaction may be reinforced by continuous repetition, making it extremely difficult to correct.

Spastic dystonia

The hemiplegic posture represents one form of what has been termed 'spastic dystonia' (Fig. 2.1).[3,6] The term is controversial given its potential confusion with extrapyramidal diseases and simply describes a sustained abnormal posture that is caused by abnormal muscle contraction. In the classical case there is a flexed, adducted, internally rotated upper limb, with a pronated forearm and flexed wrist and fingers. The lower limb is extended, internally rotated, adducted, plantarflexed and inverted at the ankle with toe flexion. This pattern is most often seen when the patient is upright. Both active muscle contraction and soft tissue changes can contribute to the abnormal postures.

In addition, there are the abnormal postures of a limb which develop during attempted movement of that limb, often involving co-contraction of agonists and antagonists. These are disordered expressions of postural synergy, which normally position and stabilise the limb in a desired position in order to carry out a local movement or task. Such background motor activity is also referred to as postural tone and abnormalities of this are a form of spastic dystonia.

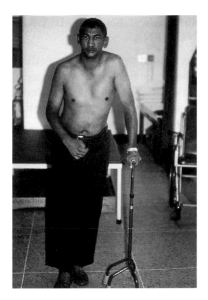

Fig 2.1 A typical hemiplegic posture of flexion and adduction in the upper limbs and extension in the lower limbs as an example of 'spastic dystonia'.

Associated reactions

Some involuntary, unnecessary activation of muscles remote from those engaged in a difficult task is a common, normal occurrence. An exaggerated form of this is seen in the UMN syndrome.[7] In a hemiplegic subject attempting to stand or walk, there may be progressive and sometimes marked flexion of the elbow. Such associated reactions can interfere with standing or walking by unbalancing the patient. Similar movement may also be provoked when lying down while making voluntary leg or foot movements or even by coughing or difficult mental activity. The reverse also occurs so that when attempting some activity with the paretic upper limb, the leg may extend or flex.

Associated reactions occur only in areas affected by an UMN lesion although there may or may not be other signs of this, such as spasticity. The severity of the associated reaction appears to be related to the difficulty of the activity provoking it. They tend to reduce when the provoking activity becomes easier to perform. Some believe that the magnitude of the associated reaction in a limb is proportional to the severity of the spasticity in the affected limb and reduces as the limb becomes less spastic.

3. Pathophysiology of spasticity

Geoffrey L. Sheean

INTRODUCTION

This book is intended to be a practical handbook of the rehabilitation of adult spasticity. Nonetheless, a thorough comprehension of its pathophysiology forms a solid foundation for clinical management, from the understanding of the clinical signs to the making of rational decisions as to the most appropriate therapy for the patient.

DEFINITION

The label 'spasticity' has been applied to many of the motor over-activities that are the positive phenomena of the upper motor neurone (UMN) syndrome (Table 1.1); true spasticity is only one of these. A very narrow definition of spasticity that is physiologically based has been given by Lance (see Chapter 2).[1]

Young[2] expanded on this definition to include more detail regarding the pathophysiology of the enhanced stretch reflex as well as the other clinical features of the UMN syndrome, both positive and negative (Table 1.1).

Spasticity and the other positive features of the UMN syndrome have in common excessive or inappropriate muscle contraction. This motor activity may be an apparently spontaneous and continuous (spastic dystonia), reflex-induced (muscle stretch, cutaneous/nociceptive stimulation). Alternatively, it may be triggered by some active movement by the patient, either locally (co-contraction), regionally (positive support reaction) or remotely (associated reaction). While the common denominator may be a lesion of the UMN, the underlying pathophysiological mechanisms of each of these phenomena have significant differences.

PATHOPHYSIOLOGY

UMNs are the neurones of any long descending tract that have a more or less direct influence upon the excitability of the lower motor neurone (anterior horn cell) either through a direct synapse (corticospinal tract) or via an interneuronal network (Table 3.1). UMNs modulate important segmental motor reflex activity in the spinal cord and the majority of the positive phenomena of the UMN syndrome arise because of interruption of the supraspinal control of these spinal reflexes. Thus, an understanding of its pathophysiology requires a discussion of these descending pathways as well as the segmental reflexes involved.

DESCENDING PATHWAYS

The role of the pyramidal tracts

The UMNs may be divided into pyramidal (those that descend through the medullary pyramids) and parapyramidal (those that do not). The word, 'parapyramidal' avoids the term 'extrapyramidal' and its association with diseases of the basal ganglia.

The UMN syndrome is frequently equated with lesions of the pyramidal tract. Thus, we talk of a 'pyramidal lesion' and a 'pyramidal pattern of weakness'. It seems that very little of the clinical UMN syndrome (Table 3.1) arises because of interruption of the pyramidal tracts.[3] Isolated lesions of the pyramidal pathways produce only mild loss of manual dexterity, an extensor plantar response and perhaps some mild hypertonia and hyperreflexia. Thus, most of the features of the UMN syndrome result from involvement of the parapyramidal tracts, some of which are in close proximity to the pyramidal tracts.

Table 3.1 Upper motor neurone pathways

- Corticospinal tract (Pyramidal tract)
- Dorsal reticulospinal tract
- Ventral reticulospinal tract
- Lateral vestibulospinal tract
- Medial vestibulospinal tract
- Rubrospinal tract
- Tectospinal tract
- Coerulospinal tract

Parapyramidal tracts (Table 3.1)

Most parapyramidal tracts arise in the brainstem, the key tracts being the dorsal reticulospinal tract (DRT), the medial reticulospinal tract (MRT) and the vestibulospinal tract (VST).[3] These descending pathways synapse upon interneuronal networks within the spinal cord that control spinal stretch reflexes, flexor reflexes and extensor reflexes. The DRT has an inhibitory influence and the other two have a predominantly excitatory influence, thus providing balanced control. In the UMN syndrome, the balance is tipped in favour of excitation. Other descending pathways are probably also involved. For example, the anti-spasticity properties of tizanidine suggest a role for the noradrenergic coerulospinal tracts, which may also be excitatory.

Descending inhibitory pathways

The dorsal reticulospinal tract arises in the ventromedial reticular formation of the brainstem, dorsal to the pyramids (Fig. 3.1). This area receives a strong facilitatory influence from the pre-motor and supplementary motor cortex via corticoreticular neurones that descend in the genu and anterior limb of the internal capsule (pyramidal fibres are posterior). There may also be some cerebellar influence. The DRT descends in the dorsolateral column of the spinal cord, just dorsal to the lateral corticospinal (pyramidal) tract. The DRT inhibits both spinal stretch reflexes and flexor reflexes.

Two important features emerge from this anatomical and functional arrangement. Firstly, the close proximity of these pathways means both the pyramidal tracts and the facilitatory corticoreticular tracts will tend to be affected by structural lesions (stroke, multiple sclerosis plaque, tumours, etc.) above the brainstem and both the pyramidal tracts and the DRT by lesions below the brainstem in the spinal cord. Such lesions will tend to produce a more complete UMN syndrome. However, because they are still anatomically separate, small structural lesions may affect only one of the tracts producing a less complete picture, as has been observed in lesions of the internal capsule.[4] The second feature is that UMN lesions above the brainstem (e.g. cortex, internal capsule), affecting the corticoreticular pathways that facilitate the DRT, will remove its cortical drive, reducing partially, but not completely, activity of the DRT. This may explain why lesions above the brainstem (cerebral) produce

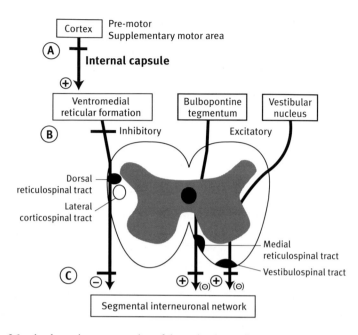

Fig. 3.1   A schematic representation of the major descending systems exerting inhibitory and excitatory supraspinal control over spinal reflex activity. The anatomical relations and the differences with respect to cortical control between the two systems means that anatomical location of the UMN lesion plays a large role in the determination of the resulting clinical pattern. **A** = lesion affecting the corticospinal fibres and the corticoreticular fibres facilitating the main inhibitory system, the dorsal reticulospinal tract. **B** = an incomplete spinal cord lesion affecting the corticospinal fibres and the dorsal reticulospinal tract. **C** = complete spinal cord lesion affecting the corticospinal fibres, dorsal reticulospinal tract and the excitatory pathways. (+) indicates an excitatory or facilitatory pathway and (–) an inhibitory pathway. The excitatory pathways have inhibitory effects on flexor reflexes. Reproduced with permission of the author from Sheean G 1995 The pathophysiology of spasticity. *Botulinum toxin in spasticity.* Meeting proceedings 26–28 October, pp 2–5.

less severe 'spasticity' than lesions of the spinal cord where complete interruptions of the DRT could occur.

Theoretically, isolated lesions of the DRT might be expected to produce spasticity without weakness. Such a picture is reminiscent of hereditary spastic paraparesis which pathologically involves the DRT with relative sparing of the corticospinal tracts.[5]

Descending excitatory pathways

The two main supraspinal excitatory pathways are the medial reticulospinal tract (MRT) and the vestibulospinal tract (VST). The MRT is probably more important in producing 'spasticity' and arises diffusely throughout the brainstem, separate from the inhibitory area described earlier. It descends in the ventromedial spinal cord, well away from the DRT and pyramidal tracts (Fig. 3.1). The excitatory pathways facilitate extensor tone and stretch reflexes, but somewhat paradoxically also appear to *inhibit* flexor reflexes; they are therefore not wholly excitatory. In contrast to the DRT, these excitatory pathways are not under cortical control. Thus, suprabulbar UMN lesions (cortex, internal capsule) will partially reduce the inhibitory influence of the DRT, tipping the balance of supraspinal control in favour of excitation by sparing the excitatory drive.

The functional responsibilities of the two systems, their separate anatomical locations and difference regarding cortical control, form the basis of the major patterns of UMN lesions — cerebral, partial (or incomplete) spinal and complete spinal. Aside from the temporal aspects of the lesion, it is largely the pattern of involvement of these systems, or more simply, the *location* of the UMN lesion rather than the aetiology of the lesion (e.g. multiple sclerosis, stroke, trauma, etc.) that determines the clinical picture. While the UMN lesion can occur anywhere along its pathway, the actual pathophysiological derangements responsible for most of the positive features of the UMN syndrome occur at the level of the spinal segments. Thus, they may all be considered 'spinal' phenomenona.

In summary, control of spinal stretch reflexes and flexor and extensor reflexes is maintained by the balance between two descending systems, one inhibitory and the other excitatory, arising in the brainstem and synapsing upon interneuronal networks within the spinal cord. The inhibitory system (DRT) is under cortical control and runs close to the pyramidal tract (dorsolateral cord). The other is not under cortical control and is located elsewhere in the ventral part of the cord. The excitatory system (MRT and VST) facilitates extensor motoneurones and stretch reflexes. The inhibitory system strongly inhibits stretch reflexes and both systems inhibit the flexor reflex afferents (FRA) responsible for flexor spasms.

SPINAL SEGMENTAL MECHANISMS

The positive features of the UMN syndrome may be divided pathophysiologically into two main groups: those that are due to disinhibited spinal reflexes and those that are not (Table 3.2). The majority are due to disinhibited spinal stretch, flexor withdrawal

Table 3.2   Pathophysiological classification of positive features of UMN syndrome

Afferent – disinhibited spinal reflexes
Stretch reflexes
    Spasticity (tonic)
    Tendon hyperreflexia (phasic)
Flexor withdrawal reflexes
    Flexor spasms
    Clasp-knife reaction (with tonic stretch reflex)
    Babinsky sign
Extensor reflexes
    Extensor spasms
    Positive support reaction

Efferent – tonic supraspinal drive?
Spastic dystonia?
Associated reactions?

and extensor reflexes. These could be classed as *afferent* mediated, meaning that sensory feedback from the affected limb initiates and maintains the motor response. Other clinical features may be *efferent* mediated, suggesting that the motor activity occurs independently of peripheral sensory feedback from the affected limb.

Spinal stretch reflexes

Phasic and tonic

A stretch reflex is a muscle contraction occurring in response to stretch of the muscle. Stretching a muscle excites the (intrafusal) muscle spindles which send impulses back to the spinal cord via large-diameter, fast-conducting sensory fibres (Ia afferents). Ia afferents carry important proprioceptive information and make a direct, monosynaptic, excitatory synapse with the α (alpha) motoneurone innervating the motor unit belonging to the extrafusal muscle fibre. This circuit is known as the stretch reflex arc (Fig. 3.2). Other muscle spindle afferents may also be important in the pathophysiology of 'spasticity' (e.g. Group II afferents). The sensitivity of the primary muscle spindle is controlled by fusimotor γ (gamma) motoneurones. Normally, the α and γ motoneurones fire together, during voluntary and involuntary (including reflex) contractions, termed 'α,γ co-activation'.

Within the spinal cord the Ia afferents make other connections through various branches to modulate their own activity, that of their own α motoneurone or that of other α motoneurones innervating the agonist or antagonist muscles. These connections involve

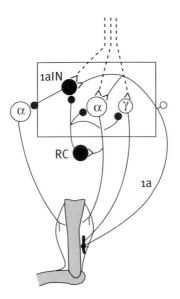

Fig. 3.2 The Ia afferent stretch reflex arc and Ia reciprocal inhibition between agonist and antagonist muscles. Both are under supraspinal control as well as segmental
regulation by Renshaw cells (RC). Reciprocal inhibition is mediated by Ia inhibitory
interneurones (Ia IN). α = alpha-motoneurones, γ = gamma motoneurones.
Reproduced with permission from the publisher, Springer-Verlag, from Hultborn H
et al 1979 On the function of recurrent inhibition in the spinal cord. Experimental
Brain Research 37: 399–403.

one (disynaptic), a few (oligosynaptic) or many (polysynaptic) inter-
posed interneurones.

Stretch reflexes are of two types according to the duration of the
stretch. Phasic stretch reflexes occur in response to very brief stretches,
such as tendon jerks elicited by a tendon tap. Tonic stretch reflexes are
produced by stretches of much longer duration, such as when testing
muscle tone clinically. Phasic stretch reflexes are predominantly, but
not exclusively monosynaptic, whereas tonic stretch reflexes are oligo-
or polysynaptic. These synapses are all under the combined inhibitory
and excitatory supraspinal control systems described earlier and the
excitability of the reflex reflects the balance of these inputs.

Normal muscle tone and postural tone

Muscle tone is the resistance felt when a joint is put passively
through its range of motion. In a normal, fully relaxed individual at

the usual speed of movement, no tonic stretch reflex is elicited, that is, no active muscle contraction is produced (Fig. 3.3). Thus, all of the resistance felt is due to the viscoelastic properties of the muscle and tendon. This calls into question reports of hypotonia, which can only come about through reduced muscle compliance and not through a reduced tonic stretch reflex.[6] The biomechanical components of hypertonia will be discussed later.

Muscle tone, as defined here, must not be confused with 'postural tone'. This well recognised motor activity,[7] also known as postural synergy, functions to stabilise or fix the limb and trunk in the optimal position for the local movement. Physiotherapists refer to both this activity, as well as to a passive resistance to movement, as 'muscle tone', which is confusing. They speak of low tone (weakness) and

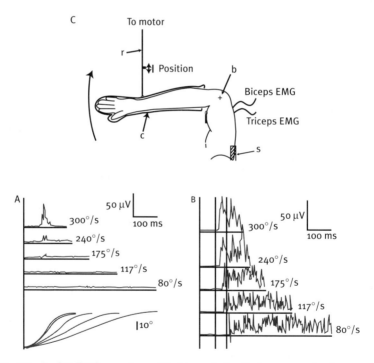

Fig. 3.3 Surface EMG recordings of the biceps during displacements of various angular velocities. **A**. Normal subjects. No EMG activity (stretch response) is elicited until very fast displacements. **B**. Spastic subjects show stretch responses at even low angular velocities, the magnitude of which increases linearly with the speed of the movement (**C**). Reproduced with permission of the publisher, Oxford University Press, from Thilmann et al 1991 The mechanism of spastic hypertonus. Brain 114: 233–244.

high tone (excessive or inappropriate muscle contraction), representing both the positive and negative phenomena of the UMN syndrome. Postural tone will be discussed more in Chapter 7.

Enhanced tonic stretch reflexes

Spasticity

Leaving aside biomechanical changes, the basis of muscle hypertonia in the UMN syndrome is spasticity, which is an enhanced tonic stretch reflex. Fig. 3.3 shows that the reflex threshold is considerably lowered in patients with spasticity; even relatively slow stretches produce a reflex response. Furthermore, tonic stretch reflexes demonstrate a linear velocity dependence, that is, the faster the movement, the greater the muscle contraction provoked. This is quite evident clinically and is due to the primary muscle spindle endings of Ia afferents being sensitive to the velocity of the stretch.

The basis of the enhanced stretch reflexes has been elucidated. The three key elements in the reflex pathway are the sensitivity of the muscle spindle (controlled by the fusimotor drive of the γ motoneurones), the intrinsic excitability of the α motoneurone, and the interneuronal processing of the Ia afferent input within the spinal cord. In short, the spindles are not more sensitive to stretch (fusimotor drive is not increased) and the α motoneurones are probably not *intrinisically* more excitable. It is the processing of the afferent information within the spinal cord that is enhanced (i.e. more excitable). The spindles and Ia afferents produce an amount of afferent input that is appropriate (not increased) for the speed and degree of stretch. Thus, when the balance of supraspinal control is tipped in favour of excitation by an UMN lesion, stretch reflexes are enhanced producing tendon hyperreflexia and spasticity.

Whether the enhanced tonic stretch reflex arises from a lowered threshold or increased gain or both is not fully resolved.[8] However, a certain velocity of movement is needed to elicit a stretch reflex. The critical angular velocity may be around 100° per second[9] although others have found thresholds as low as 40° per second.[10, 11] The existence of a critical velocity is important for three reasons. Firstly, it emphasises that spasticity is due to an enhanced *kinetic* stretch reflex; it is not present without movement and once the movement ceases there is no spasticity. Secondly, mild degrees of spasticity may be missed unless the movement is rapid enough. Thirdly, the question of whether active movement of an agonist is constrained by spasticity in the antagonist will depend upon the speed of the stretching movement. Although this has been observed,[12] patients with UMN lesions tend to move slowly, perhaps too slowly, to elicit spasticity in the antagonist.[13]

Despite their enhancement at rest, tonic stretch reflexes are said to be normal when the 'spastic' muscles are actively contracting.[14] The lack of spasticity during active contraction is difficult to detect clinically.

Static stretch reflexes

As mentioned, spasticity is chiefly a kinetic stretch reflex evoked by a critical velocity of movement and is said to have only a minimal static component.[15] However, one often sees continuing muscle contraction (on EMG) when the stretch is maintained, even though movement has stopped.[16] This suggests the presence of an enhanced *static* stretch response, possibly mediated by static responsive spindle endings (Group II) whose firing is length dependent.[14] True spasticity, with a superimposable velocity-dependent dynamic stretch response, may co-exist.

A static stretch response may sometimes diminish and disappear completely (on EMG) if the stretch is maintained for several minutes. Thereafter, tone may be normal in a previously markedly hypertonic muscle and no stretch response can be initiated, even with very rapid stretches. Physiotherapists have long known that stretching can reduce spasticity as well as the soft tissue changes of muscle stiffness, but only for a short time; it quickly returns if the length is not maintained by splinting.[17]

Hypertonia in UMN lesions

The role of biomechanical changes

In addition to the appearance of neural factors (e.g. spasticity), the biomechanical contribution to muscle tone may also become pathologically increased in UMN lesions. Muscles (and tendons) may become stiff and less compliant and can ultimately develop fixed contractures. These secondary soft tissue changes presumably occur as a result of muscles not being placed through a normal range of movement through either weakness (and poor positioning) or excessive but abnormal contraction (e.g. sustained flexor spasms); both leave the muscle in a shortened position for prolonged periods.

Recognition that muscle tone is the additive result of these two different components, neural and biomechanical, is central to the understanding and management of patients with UMN lesions; both factors clearly require different therapeutic approaches. Secondary joint changes, frozen shoulder and heterotopic ossification will also limit movement.

At some joints, such as the ankle, reduced muscle compliance may account for most or all of the hypertonia and reduced range of movement.[18] It will restrict movement even at slow speeds because this kind of resistance is not dependent upon the velocity of the stretch. Thus, in reality the biomechanical component of hypertonia may be far more important than pathologically enhanced stretch reflexes in opposing movement.

This increase in muscles stiffness may partly involve changes in their connective tissue[19] as well as a kind of stiffness within the muscle fibre itself, known as thixotropy. Thixotropy in engineering describes a dynamic viscosity of fluids. For example, initially upon stirring paint it feels thick and stiff but then becomes much easier to stir after one has broken down links between the paint molecules. If left to stand, the paint 'sets' and again becomes difficult to stir.

A similar phenomenon in muscle fibres has been attributed to abnormal cross-bridges between actin and myosin muscle filaments. Muscles left at a certain length develop these cross-bridges resulting in a short-term stiffness that can be quickly worked out by repetitive lengthening of the muscle. It has been suggested that thixotropy is increased in spasticity.[20] Marked hypertonia following a strong isotonic contraction of a muscle that can be worked out by repeated stretching and that is not associated with significant EMG activity is probably due to pathologically enhanced thixotropy.

Reduced muscle compliance may precede the development of muscle contracture. Contracture is an essentially irreversible shortening of a muscle due to a reduced number of sarcomeres[21] whereas reduced compliance may be due to a remodelling of the muscle connective tissue.[19] Although they often occur together, muscle tone within a range of movement reduced by contracture may sometimes be normal. Recently, the association between contractures and reduced muscle compliance has been emphasised whilst highlighting a poor correlation between contracture and spasticity (as a hyperexcitable tonic stretch reflex).[22]

Tendon hyperreflexia and clonus

Although tendon hyperreflexia arises through very similar mechanisms to that of spasticity, several observations suggest that phasic and tonic stretch reflexes are controlled somewhat differently. Firstly, tendon hyperreflexia and spasticity may occur independently. Secondly, clinical electrophysiological correlations show a dissociation between the two.[23] Thirdly, each may be affected independently by certain medications; baclofen reduces spasticity without significantly altering tendon reflexes. Finally, patients with pathological states (e.g. hyperthyroidism) and some healthy nervous subjects can have extremely brisk tendon reflexes but no spasticity.

Clonus can also be seen in normal subjects and is a variant of tendon hyperreflexia. Clonus does not occur without exaggerated tendon jerks and provides no more diagnostic information. The mechanism is simple. A brisk stretch of the gastrocnemius–soleus (rapid dorsiflexion of the ankle) elicits a stretch reflex, the gastrocnemius–soleus contracts, plantarflexing the ankle and eliminating the stretch, and the muscle relaxes. If this relaxation is rapid enough, while the examiner maintains a continued stretching force, another stretch reflex will be elicited and the ankle will again plantarflex and so forth. A rhythmic, tremor-like pattern of contraction and relaxation is set up. This will generally continue for as long as the dorsiflexion force is maintained by the examiner, producing sustained clonus. However, the persistence of clonus simply reflects the degree of gain of the stretch reflex pathway and unsustained clonus can also occur in UMN lesions. Burke[6] notes that much of the eliciting and maintaining of clonus lies in the skilled technique of the examiner.

Another clinical corollary is reflex radiation described in the last chapter. Muscle spindles are sensitive to vibration and a tendon tap sets up a wave of vibration that spreads further afield, exciting spindles in other muscles and producing phasic stretch reflexes (jerks). Again reflex radiation provides no new information except to demonstrate the degree of the heightened stretch reflexes.

Clasp-knife phenomenon

Length dependency of the tonic stretch reflex

The clasp-knife phenonemon is essentially a variant of spasticity. A rapid joint movement stretches a muscle and elicits a velocity-dependent tonic stretch reflex. The resistance produced by the reflex contraction of this muscle slows the movement, thus reducing the stimulus for the stretch reflex to below the velocity threshold. The muscle contraction therefore stops, fairly abruptly, allowing the examiner who is keeping up the tension to continue the movement with minimal resistance.

The clasp-knife phenomenon is best observed in the quadriceps muscles where there is an additional mechanism. Tonic stretch reflex sensitivity here is not only velocity dependent but also length dependent. In lower limb extensors (quadriceps and gastrocnemius–soleus), reflex sensitivity is *decreased* by lengthening. In contrast, the stretch reflex in flexor muscles (hamstrings, tibialis anterior) is *increased* by lengthening. The opposite pattern occurs in the upper limbs in cerebral palsy.[24] So, as the examiner is flexing the knee, the velocity of the movement is being slowed by the reflex contraction of the quadriceps at the same time as its length is increasing — both factors are acting to reduce the sensitivity of the reflex. A critical point is reached whereby the velocity is too slow and the length of the quadriceps too long to sustain a stretch reflex and the quadriceps contraction opposing the movement ceases to cause the 'give way' effect. The length-dependent inhibition continues and prevents reactivation of the tonic stretch reflex as the movement continues, unopposed.

The length-dependent sensitivity of the tonic stretch reflex in the quadriceps is due to active inhibition of the reflex. Previously, inhibitory Ib afferents from the golgi tendon organs were thought to be responsible. The golgi tendon organs supposedly suddenly fired when the tension produced by the stretch reflex became too great, as a kind of protective mechanism. However, golgi tendon organs actually fire at low muscle tensions and stop firing once the active contraction stops. Furthermore, Ib non-reciprocal inhibition is actually reduced in many hemiplegic patients with spasticity.[25] The golgi tendon organs therefore contribute little if anything at all to the clasp-knife phenomenon.

Instead, the inhibition of the quadriceps stretch reflex is mediated by flexor reflex afferents (FRAs). FRAs inhibit extensors (e.g. quadriceps) and facilitate flexors (e.g. hamstrings) and are responsible for the normal flexor withdrawal reflexes and the flexor spasms of the UMN syndrome. Thus, the clasp-knife phenomenon represents an overlap between two major pathophysiological mechanisms in the UMN syndrome, disinhibition of tonic stretch reflexes and disinhibition of flexor reflexes. One might expect to see the quadriceps clasp-knife phenomenon in association with flexor spasms but this is not always the case.

Flexor spasms

Flexor spasms chiefly affect the lower limbs, typically consisting of simultaneous flexion of the hip, knee and ankle (dorsiflexion). Although they may appear to occur spontaneously, flexor spasms are reflex contractions occurring in response to a variety of sensory stimuli, including cutaneous and nociceptive stimuli and bladder or bowel distension or irritation (e.g. catheter, urinary infections). These effects are mediated by the FRAs, which are 'multi-modal' and include Group II spindle afferents and Group II, III and IV non-encapsulated mechanoreceptors in muscles and joint. They have in common their ability to evoke a flexion reflex. Very severe flexor spasms may be accompanied by emptying of the bowels and bladder (mass reflex action).

FRA connections to the motoneurones are polysynaptic and under supraspinal control. Most of the supraspinal inhibition comes via the DRT, but alo from the medial reticulospinal tracts (MRT) and vestibulospinal tracts (VST).[3] The rubrospinal and corticospinal tracts facilitate FRAs. Thus, a partial or 'incomplete' spinal cord lesion involving the DRT and sparing the MRT and VST will produce only moderate flexor spasms. A complete spinal cord lesion affecting all three tracts leaves the FRAs totally without supraspinal inhibition and very severe flexor spasms are the rule ('paraplegia-in-flexion'). Furthermore, a cerebral UMN lesion may remove the cortical facilitation of the DRT but the continuing DRT output and the intact MRT and VST are usually sufficient to prevent flexor spasms. The clasp-knife phenomenon may still occur, however.

Flexor spasms are due to disinhibition of the normal flexor withdrawal reflex. During normal motor development this reflex comes under supraspinal control to take part in walking and to protect the foot when a painful stimulus is encountered. The extensor plantar response (Babinsky sign) is also a disinhibited flexor withdrawal reflex, but has some added complexities.[6]

Extensor spasms

Partial spinal cord lesions may destroy the DRT but spare the MRT and VST. All three tend to inhibit FRAs (produce flexor spasms) but the latter two also facilitate extensor motoneurones. Thus, both flexor and extensor spasms may occur but the latter tend to predominate (paraplegia-in-extension). Stimuli to extensor spasms include non-painful (non-nociceptive) cutaneous stimuli to certain areas (e.g. groin, buttock and posterior aspect of leg), body movement (especially with iliopsoas stretch), a flexion withdrawal reflex in the opposite limb (a crossed extensor reflex utilised by the stepping generator in the spinal cord to produce the cyclical movements of walking) and assuming the upright posture (a vestibular postural reflex). The latter physiologically increases vestibulospinal drive to anti-gravity muscles. Leg extension may also be seen as part of an associated reaction occurring with upper limb activity. Even though extensor tone and spasms may dominate the clinical picture, stimulation of the partially disinhibited FRAs by ulcers, bedsores, urinary tract infections, constipation etc. may turn paraplegia-in-extension into paraplegia-in-flexion.

The positive support reaction has been attributed to an extensor reflex triggered by the sensory feedback (cutaneous/proprioceptive) of the ball of the foot touching the floor. This may represent the disinhibition of the physiological positive supporting reflex ('standing reflex') seen in infants and animals.[14]

Co-contraction

Simultaneous contraction of agonist and antagonist (co-contraction) is an important component of normal reciprocal innervation.[26] It is required for many normal human movements, providing postural fixation or stabilisation, and can be activated and de-activated as the movement demands. Thus, it is a motor activity which is purposeful, dynamic or responsive, and functional, forming part of the normal postural synergy. In the UMN syndrome (and dystonia), agonist and antagonist muscles may co-contract inappropriately and be dysfunctional. Co-contraction could restrict movement of the agonist and contribute to its apparent weakness[27] but its role in the impairment of movement in the UMN syndrome has been questioned.[13,28] For the ankle, biomechanical changes in gastrocnemius–soleus may be more restrictive to dorsiflexion than any active contraction.[13]

Co-contraction is activated and de-activated at a cortical level.[29] Modulation of co-contraction also occurs at a spinal level by a process of Ia reciprocal inhibition (Fig. 3.3); Ia spindle afferent activity inhibits, via an interneurone, the α motorneurone of the antagonist (and vice versa). Renshaw cell regulation is also involved. This segmental activity is under supraspinal control and is impaired in both spasticity and dystonia.

True co-contraction should be distinguished from a tonic stretch reflex. Active dorsiflexion of the ankle may stretch the triceps surae and elicit a tonic stretch reflex.[12] This reflex response would normally be suppressed by Ia reciprocal inhibition from the contraction of tibialis anterior. In contrast, true co-contraction will occur when the contractions are *isometric*, in the absence of any stretching movement.

A corollary of this is that excessive contraction of an antagonist (either spasm or reflex induced), in the presence of retained reciprocal inhibition, could inhibit activity in the agonist, contributing further to its apparent weakness. Some workers have shown that reciprocal inhibition from soleus to tibialis anterior is preserved in spastic patients.[30] Thus, attempted ankle dorsiflexion could result in co-contraction of triceps surae, as well as a tonic stretch reflex, which would mechanically oppose the dorsiflexion. In addition, the active contraction of soleus by these two mechanisms could actively inhibit firing of tibialis anterior (by Ia reciprocal inhibition) adding to the apparent weakness of tibialis anterior. In support of this notion, blockade of the triceps surae afferent fibres led to increased strength in the ankle dorsiflexors.[31]

Associated reactions

The phenomenon of motor effort in one part of the body being associated with unintentional motor activity elsewhere was described in Chapter 2. These associated reactions have also been described as 'radiation' of voluntary efforts.[27] Although long recognised[7] they have not been well studied. The degree of the associated reaction appears to correlate with the degree of effort being expended elsewhere and also with the degree of hypertonia in the limb demonstrating the associated reaction; this hypertonia does not necessarily equate with spasticity (i.e. hyperactive stretch reflexes). Recently, Dickstein and colleagues[32] studied the associated reaction of elbow flexion during walking. They found that although contraction of the elbow flexors was required to produce the movement, the elbow flexion was maintained by soft tissue stiffness of the muscles rather than by active muscle contraction.

Associated reactions may represent one of the efferent-mediated phenomena of the UMN syndrome mentioned earlier. The pathophysiology of the tonic drive to the α motoneurones is unknown and possible mechanisms have been reviewed elsewhere.[32]

Spastic dystonia

This term is used to describe the abnormal posture present in the patient with the UMN syndrome,[2] including the 'hemiplegic posture'. Abnormal postures may be produced by soft tissue changes, including contractures, but also by continuous (active) muscle contraction. This phenomenon is fundamentally different to spasticity in several ways.[6] Firstly, spasticity is a kinetic or dynamic stretch reflex, dependent upon afferent feedback from movement of the stretched muscle. In contrast, the muscle contraction of spastic dystonia continues in the absence of movement and is not abolished by dorsal root section. Thus, spastic dystonia is not dependent upon afferent input from the limb and is thus not a *reflex*, as such. It is, however, susceptible to the modulating effects of posture, presumably through vestibular mechanisms. It may be considered a form of *efferent* muscular hyperactivity, dependent upon continuous supraspinal drive to the α motoneurones.[6] The distinction between the 'efferent' spastic dystonia and the 'afferent' muscular hyperactivities, such as spasticity, is clearly important from a therapeutic point of view. Medications and surgical procedures designed to dampen spinal stretch reflexes and flexor reflexes will not be effective in controlling the non-reflex mediated spastic dystonia.

The abnormal stereotypic movement patterns characteristic of hemiplegia may also be considered a form of spastic dystonia — abnormal postures evoked by movement. Abnormalities of postural synergy ('postural tone'), associated reactions and abnormal co-contraction could be included in this group. The inhibitory activity of Renshaw cells appears to be under control by reticulospinal systems (similar to stretch and flexor reflexes) and may play a role here.[33]

ELECTROPHYSIOLOGICAL STUDIES

Many electrophysiological tests of spinal reflex activity have been studied in order to understand better the pathophysiological mechanisms of spasticity and allied phenomena.[34] The most useful involve spinal inhibitory mechanisms and flexor reflexes.

Segmental inhibitory mechanisms

Four inhibitory mechanisms within the spinal cord have been studied in patients with spasticity: Ia pre-synaptic inhibition, Ia reciprocal inhibition, Ib non-reciprocal inhibition and Renshaw cell

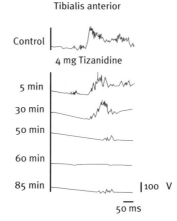

Tibialis anterior

Fig. 3.4   Flexor withdrawal reflexes (surface EMG) recorded from the tibialis anterior of a patient with spasticity after electrical stimulation of the sural nerve. Note the marked reduction in the reflex after tizanidine is administered. From Delawaide and Pennisi.[25] Reproduced with permission from Advanstar Communications Inc. as reprinted from Neurology®, Nov. 1994, Vol (#44), Number (#11), Supplement (#9), and page (#S21–S28). Neurology® is a registered trademark of the American Academy of Neurology.

PLASTICITY

The period of 'shock' is said to be due to the sudden loss of supraspinal control and does not occur in slowly developing lesions.[6] The delayed and slow emergence of the positive features is taken as evidence that they are not merely due to the simple unbalancing of inhibition and excitation but involve some functional or structural rearrangement of the central nervous system (CNS). Furthermore, spasticity may decline with time. The exact mechanisms of this CNS plasticity are unknown but could involve collateral sprouting and changes in receptor sensitivity.[3]

CONCLUSION

The pathophysiology of spasticity and the other positive features of the upper motor neurone syndrome continues to be a complex and incompletely understood area. Nonetheless, knowledge of the basic concepts presented in this chapter will facilitate interpretation of the clinical signs and allow more rationale therapy. Some of the important concepts are the minimal role played by the pyramidal tract, the dual inhibitory and excitatory supraspinal systems controlling the segmental spinal reflex activity that produces most of these positive phenomena, the major role that the site of the UMN lesion plays in producing the clinical picture as opposed to the aetiology, and the importance of secondary soft tissue changes. The fact that many of the clinical features are due to separate pathophysiological mechanisms means that while they may commonly occur together, they may also be seen independently and may respond differently to medications. There are a number of electrophysiological tests of spinal reflex activity that have been found to be abnormal in the UMN syndrome, some of which may correlate with the degree of spasticity. However, none are abnormal consistently in all patients leaving one to question their pathophysiological role and suggest that spasticity may be a pathophysiologically heterogeneous entity. Thus, we are a long way from directing medications at the patient's profile of electrophysiological test abnormalities and their putative neurotransmitters. Much more work is needed in the areas of electrophysiology, neurochemistry and neuronal plasticity to complete the picture.

REFERENCES

1. Lance JW 1980 Symposium synopsis. In: Feldman RG, Young RR, Koella WP (eds) Spasticity: disordered motor control. Year Book Medical Publishers, Chicago, pp 485–494
2. Young RR 1994 Spasticity: a review. Neurology 44 (suppl 9): S12–S20
3. Brown P 1994 Pathophysiology of spasticity (editorial). J Neurol Neurosurg Psychiatry 57: 773–777
4. Fries W, Danek A, Scheidtman K, Hamburger C. Motor recovery following capsular stroke. Role of descending pathways from multiple motor areas. Brain 1993; 116: 369–382
5. Chou SM 1992 Pathology — light microscopy of amyotrophic lateral sclerosis. In: Smith RA (ed) Handbook of amyotrophic lateral sclerosis. Marcel Dekker, New York, pp 133–181
6. Burke D 1988 Spasticity as an adaptation to pyramidal tract injury. In: Waxman SG (ed) Advances in Neurology: Functional Recovery in Neurological Disease Vol 47 Raven Press, New York, pp 401–423
7. Walshe FMR 1923 On certain tonic or postural reflexes in hemiplegia, with special reference to the so-called 'associated movements'. Brain 46: 1–37
8. Noth J 1991 Trends in the pathophysiology and pharmacotherapy of spasticity. J Neurol 238: 131–139
9. Burke D, Gillies JD, Lance JW 1970 The quadriceps stretch reflex in human spasticity. J Neurol Neurosurg Psychiatry 33: 216–223
10. Powers RK, Marder-Meyer OT, Rymer WZ 1988 Quantitative relations between hypertonia and stretch reflex threshold in spastic hemiparesis. Ann Neurol 23: 115–124
11. Powers RK, Campbell DL, Rymer WZ 1989 Stretch reflex dynamics in spastic elbow flexors. Ann Neurol 25: 32–42
12. Corcos DM, Gottlieb GL, Penn RD, Myklebust B, Agarwal GC 1986 Movement deficits caused by hyperexcitable stretch reflexes in spastic humans. Brain 109: 1043–1058
13. Dietz V, Quintern J, Berger W 1981 Electrophysiological studies of gait in spasticity and rigidity. Evidence that altered mechanical properties of muscle contribute to hypertonia. Brain 104: 431–449
14. Rothwell JC 1994 Control of human voluntary movement. 2nd edition. Chapman and Hall, London

15. Burke D, Knowles L, Andrews C, Ashby P 1972 Spasticity, decerebrate rigidity and the clasp knife phenomenon. An experimental study in the cat. Brain 95: 31–48
16. Denny-Brown D 1980 Preface: Historical aspects of the relation of spasticity to movement. In: Feldman RG, Young RR, Koella WP (eds) Spasticity: disordered motor control. Year Book Medical Publishers, Chicago, pp 1–15
17. Tremblay F, Malouin F, Richards CL, Dumas F 1990 Effects of prolonged muscle stretch on reflex and voluntary muscle activations in children with spastic cerebral palsy. Scand J Rehabil Med 22: 171–180
18. Dietz V, Berger W 1983 Normal and impaired regulation of muscle stiffness in gait: a new hypothesis about muscle hypertonia. Exp Neurol 79: 680–687
19. Goldspink G, Williams PE 1990 Muscle fibre and connective tissue changes associated with use and disuse. In: Ada A, Canning C (eds) Foundations for practice. Topics in neurological physiotherapy. Heinemann, London, pp 197–218
20. Carey JR 1990 Manual stretch: effect on finger movement control in stroke subjects with spastic extrinsic finger flexor muscles. Arch Phys Med Rehabil 71: 888–894
21. Tardieu C, Huet de la Tour E, Bret MD, Tardieu G 1982 Muscle hypoextensibility in children with cerebral palsy: I. Clinical and experimental observations. Arch Phys Med Rehabil 63: 97–102
22. O'Dwyer NJ, Ada L, Neilson PD 1996 Spasticity and muscle contracture following stroke. Brain 119: 1737–1749
23. Delwaide PJ, Gerrard P 1993 Reduction of non-reciprocal (Ib) inhibition: a key factor for determining spastic muscle stiffness. International Congress on Stroke Rehabilitation, Berlin
24. Andrews CJ, Neilson PD, Knowles L 1973 Electromyographic study of the rigido-spasticity of athetosis. J Neurol Neurosurg Psychiatry 36: 94–103
25. Delwaide PJ and Pennisi G. Tizanidine and electrophysiologic analysis of spinal control mechanisms in humans with spasticity. Neurology 44 (suppl 9): S21–S28
26. Basmajian JV 1978 Muscles alive. Their functions revealed by electromyography. 4th edition. Williams and Wilkins, Baltimore
27. Weisendanger M 1990 Weakness and the upper motor neurone syndrome: a critical pathophysiological appraisal. In: Berardelli A, Benecke R, Manfredi M, Marsden CD (eds) Motor Disturbances II. Academic Press, London, pp 319–331
28. Fellows SJ, Klaus C, Ross HF, Thilmann AF 1994 Agonist and antagonist EMG activation during isometric torque development at the elbow in spastic hemiparesis. Electroenceph Clin Neurophysiol 93: 106–112
29. Humphrey DR, Reed DJ 1983 Separate cortical systems for control of joint movement and joint stiffness: reciprocal activation and coactivation of antagonist muscles. In: Desmedt JE (ed). Motor control mechanisms in health and disease. Raven Press, New York, pp 347–372
30. Yanagisawa N, Tanaka R, Ito Z 1976 Reciprocal Ia inhibition in spastic hemiplegia of man. Brain 99: 555–574
31. Yanagisawa N, Tanaka R 1978 Reciprocal Ia inhibition in spastic paralysis in man. Electroenceph Clin Neurophysiol (suppl) 34: 521–526
32. Dickstein R, Heffes Y, Abulaffio N 1996 Electromyographic and positional changes in the elbows of spastic hemiparetic patients during walking. Electroenceph Clin Neurophysiol 101: 491–496
33. Mazzocchio R, Rossi A 1997 Involvement of spinal recurrent inhibition in spasticity. Further insight into the regulation of Renshaw cell activity. Brain 120: 991–1003
34. Delwaide PJ, Olivier E 1987 Pathophysiological aspects of spasticity in man. In: Benecke R, Conrad B, Marsden CD (eds) Motor Disturbaces I. Academic Press, London, pp 153–167
35. Shahani BT, Young RR 1980 The flexor reflex in spasticity. In: Feldman RG, Young RR, Koella WP (eds) Spasticity: disordered motor control. Year Book Medical Publishers, Chicago, pp 287–295
36. Thilmann AF, Fellows SJ, Garms E 1991 The mechanism of spastic muscle hypertonus. Brain 114: 233–244

4. Clinical rating of spasticity

Davina Richardson

INTRODUCTION

In a survey of health professionals working in the field of neurology, 94% of respondents felt that it was important to measure spasticity, but only 39% made attempts to do so in practice.[1] As the forthcoming chapter on treatment goals and outcome measures will emphasise, being able to measure spasticity is invaluable in assessing the response to treatment.

The clinical measurement of spasticity is a 'difficult and unresolved problem',[2] partly because of its complex and multifactorial nature. There is no definitive clinical measurement of spasticity which is valid, sensitive and reliable. Current research is focusing on improving objective measurement and the development of new tools for the direct or indirect clinical evaluation of spasticity.

As discussed in Chapter 2, spasticity is only one of the positive features of the upper motor neurone (UMN) syndrome and cannot be viewed in isolation.[3,4] Clinical measurement of the other positive features of the UMN syndrome is also difficult, although spasm rating scales have been developed[5] and clonus can be evaluated by the number of beats.[6]

This chapter will therefore concentrate on clinical measurement of spasticity alone and is divided into three sections. Section one will focus on the direct measurement of spasticity using resistance to passive movement and range of joint motion. Section two will address the indirect measurement of spasticity by evaluation of the consequences of spasticity. Finally, section three will briefly mention measures of spasticity that are useful in clinical trials. Electromyographic assessment of spasticity is also a valuable clinical tool; this is discussed further in Chapter 9.

SECTION ONE

DIRECT MEASUREMENT OF SPASTICITY

Before describing methods of clinical rating of spasticity, it is important to emphasise its highly variable nature. Spasticity is influenced by the position of the limb against gravity, the degree of co-contraction of the antagonist muscle, the extent of available voluntary control in the limb, the presence of noxious stimuli, constipation, the state of the bladder and the time since the patient last had medication (Table 4.1).[7] In addition, non-neurological factors, such as the time of day, ambient temperature, fatigue, emotion and mood, and the patient's mental state should be considered; for example, marked hypertonia in a clinic or hospital may be much better at home. Clinicians should remember the multifactorial and fluctuating nature of spasticity when drawing conclusions from the measurements. This is particularly important in making the decision to treat spasticity and in judging response to treatment.

Spasticity manifests clinically as hypertonia. Thus, the degree of resistance to passive movement (tone) and available range of movement in a limb provide some measure of spasticity. However, these measures include both neural (spasticity) and non-neural (biomechanical) components.[8,9] A simple clinical measure of resistance to passive movement and range of movement cannot reliably distinguish between the two and so cannot always give a valid representation of true spasticity. This is especially important in the evaluation of treatments which only influence the neural component of tone, e.g. anti-spastic drugs. Bearing this in mind, let us now proceed to discuss the measures available.

Table 4.1   Factors influencing hypertonia in the UMN syndrome

Factors tending to increase tone	Factors that may reduce tone
Noxious stimuli	Good health
Fatigue	Well rested
Speed of movement (fast)	Slow movement
Constipation	Normal bowel
Bladder infection/need to empty	Well-controlled bladder
Fear/anxiety	Happy
Degree of co-contraction of antagonist	Comfortable position; well supported
Tone of voice	Medication levels
General comfort	
Mental state/emotional state	
Temperature of the room (cold or hot)	Temperature of the room or muscle itself

MEASUREMENT OF RESISTANCE TO PASSIVE MOVEMENT (MUSCLE TONE)

Ashworth Scale

The benchmark spasticity rating scale is the Ashworth Scale, in its original[10] or modified forms.[11] The original Ashworth Scale was developed for a study of an oral anti-spastic agent in the treatment of spasticity in adults with multiple sclerosis (Table 4.2). It was later modified to incorporate a '1+' rating (Table 4.2) and found to have good reliability for elbow flexor tone.[11] Similar results from other studies[12,13] would indicate that, although the Ashworth scale is not perfect, when combined with the patients' accounts of their symptoms and the effects of the spasticity on their motor function it can provide useful information.

Whether one should use the modified or the original Ashworth Scale is debatable. A study comparing the inter-rater reliability of each found little difference between them.[14] Both scales were unreliable for the measurement of tone in the lower limb (ankle), but reliable in the upper limb (elbow).

One considerable drawback of the Ashworth Scale, which has not been addressed, is the lack of standardisation of technique in performing the tone measurements. The velocity of the passive movement could be standardised by matching the movement to a verbal cadence (saying 'one thousand and one' as you move the limb). Standardising the testing position to supine and allowing the patient time to accommodate to this position may also be useful. Whether one should do repetitive movements of the limb is debatable as these may modify stretch reflexes and influence the more dynamic biomechanical properties of the muscle, such as thixotropy (see Chapter 3). In practice, one movement from a

Table 4.2   The modified Ashworth Scale of spasticity[11]

0	No increase in tone
1	Slight increase in tone giving a 'catch' when the limb was moved in flexion or extension
1+*	Slight increase in muscle tone, manifested by a catch, followed by minimal resistance throughout the remainder (less than half) of the ROM
2	More marked increase in tone but the limb easily flexed
3	Considerable increase in tone, passive movement difficult
4	Limb rigid in flexion or extension

*The original Ashworth Scale did not include a 1+ rating. ROM = range of movement.

position of rest should be sufficient to score on the Ashworth Scale. It should also be possible to standardise the force applied in moving the limb. Resolving these issues may well improve the scale's usefulness.

For the measurement of spasticity involving multiple muscles, a composite Ashworth Scale score has been used. In paraplegia, a score is given for hip flexion and abduction, knee flexion and extension, and ankle dorsiflexion for each leg; the scores are added and the total divided by ten to arrive at an average grade.[15,16] This method has not been validated nor its reliability tested but it could be useful where spasticity is not isolated to a single muscle, which is often the case.

Advantages and disadvantages

The advantages of the Ashworth Scale are that it is simple, easy to use and its results are easily communicated. It is used widely in clinical practice and research, and is well known. The Scale has been shown to correlate with other more reliable measures of spasticity such as torque and electromyography (EMG) measurements during ramp and hold angular displacements.[17]

The disadvantages of the Ashworth Scale include the fact that it measures the combined effects of both biomechanical and neural components of tone. Performance parameters are difficult to standardise. The zero point is ambiguous and the modified scale has been criticised because it may not be ordinal. Finally, there is relatively limited data on the inter-trial and inter-rater reliability of the Scale's use in a large variety of muscle groups and joints. These criticisms also apply to range of movement measurements (see below).

If the user is aware of the shortcomings of the Ashworth Scale and does not attempt excessive statistical analysis of the data, then it has some value in communicating the degree of spasticity to other clinicians.

Other means of clinically evaluating tone include observer rating scales, such as a simple three point scale of mild, moderate or severe, or a four point scale, as in the Motor Assessment Scale, designed for the evaluation of disability in stroke.[18] Reliability studies of the total Motor Assessment Scale have found the item on tone to be less reliable than the other eight items.

RANGE OF MOVEMENT

Goniometry

In the UMN syndrome, joint range is influenced not only by spasticity, but also by joint disease, heterotopic ossification, pain and the non-neural, biomechanical factors within the muscle itself.[19] Measurement of joint range is performed most commonly by a hand-held goniometer. From a number of studies of the reliability and validity of this measurement technique,[20,21] the conclusions are that:

1. Repeated testing by the same rater is more reliable than testing using different raters[22]
2. Reliability of measurements is joint specific, perhaps even movement specific[23]
3. The medical condition of the subject influences the reliability of measurements.[24]

Despite this, the literature is undecided on whether an accurate recording of joint range can be made using a goniometer. It seems that reliability is best for large single-plane movement joints and is improved if a single person performs the measures. Standardised positions and normal values are available for all joints,[25] making reliability somewhat better.

In practice, measurement of a joint angle in a subject with spasticity is difficult. It is best carried out by two people; one to hold the limb and the second to position the goniometer correctly. Use of standardised recording sheets assists the accuracy and interpretation of the angle on the instrument. For example, a neutral plantar grade position of the ankle may be recorded as 90 degrees dorsiflexion or as 0 degrees, or an extended elbow as 180 degrees extension or 0 degrees. The force applied to the limb may also influence the reading of the joint angle; a force of 100 mm Hg may record a very different joint angle than when a 200 mm Hg force is applied. Attempts to standardise the force have been made using the hand-held myometer or a modified sphygmomanometer.[26]

OTHER MEASURES OF RESISTANCE TO PASSIVE MOVEMENT AND JOINT RANGE

The following techniques are used more in the research or laboratory setting and are therefore somewhat less useful to the practising clinician.

Pendulum test (Wartenburg test)

The Wartenburg test is a biomechanical measure of the resistance to passive stretch.[27] It has only been studied for the quadriceps muscle and is not suitable for any other muscle groups. With the patient lying in the supine position, the measured leg is dropped from full extension and allowed to swing freely. The amplitude, frequency and number of swings are recorded with an electrogoniometer. Spastic legs have a reduced number and amplitude of swings, which can be described mathematically.

Isokinetics

Isokinetic measurement and torque generators provide useful, repeatable and reliable information about the state of the limb and its resistance to passive movement.[28] Limbs fixed to a torque generator are moved to quantify the amount of torque (amount of force induced by moving the limb over a certain angle) and/or threshold. A variety of devices are available with good inter-rater reliability.[29] Some apparatus appear to be able to overcome the problem of interference of mechanical muscle properties and measure only the increase in tone.[30] This enables quantification of phasic and tonic reflex activity of a spastic muscle.[17] This equipment is expensive and not readily available to most people in the clinic.

Myometry

Resistance of a joint to passive movements can also be measured with hand-held myometers. This means of rating spasticity is perhaps underused as the myometer is portable and easily available. The technique is non-invasive, easy to learn, quick and easy to carry out and, after the initial outlay, the machines cost little to maintain. Standardised positions for myometry are available. Malouin and colleagues[31] concluded that the reliability of spasticity measurements by a hand-held dynamometer is dependent upon the joint being tested (i.e. high reliability for the elbow flexors and less reliable assessment of the plantar flexors), similar to the Ashworth Scale. They also noted lower reliability when tone was high. In practice, one might therefore limit the use of myometry to the single-plane upper limb joints of moderate spasticity, similar to the Ashworth Scale.

SECTION TWO

MEASUREMENT OF COMMON CONSEQUENCES OF SPASTICITY AND OTHER POSITIVE FEATURES OF THE UMN SYNDROME

Another approach to the assessment of spasticity, commonly used when evaluating treatment outcome, is to measure some of the clinical consequences of spasticity. These include:

1. Pain
2. Abnormal posturing of a limb (spastic dystonia)
3. Associated reactions
4. Difficulty generating force in the antagonist muscle group
5. Reduced functional ability.

Great care needs to be taken when interpreting data from such scales as few have undergone rigorous testing due to the novelty of the presentation. Another caution is the assumption that spasticity is the cause of the clinical problems. This may not be so as many of these problems are multifactorial, especially functional impairment.

Pain measurement

A commonly used tool to measure pain is the visual analogue scale.[32] In order to be useful the scale needs to be administered carefully, particularly when making comparisons between before and after treatment.[33] However, it may be too unstable and imprecise to be used as a measure of clinically significant change. Therefore, visual analogue scales should be only one part of a total system for grading spasticity. In practice, many neurological patients are incapable of using the scale and the carer or therapist may be more suitable. Some subjects seem to respond better if they are given a pain rating scale. In a global pain rating scale, patients rate their pain from 0–100, where 0 is no pain and 100 is the worst possible pain. Obviously both means of studying pain rely on the patient understanding an abstract concept of pain.

Video, photography and the Physician Rating Scale

Abnormal limb posturing may have a variety of causes in the UMN syndrome, including spasticity, and may be measured in several ways. Goniometry and written descriptions have their limitations. The Physician Clinical Rating Scale of video or photographic recordings relies on accurate analysis of the patient performing a series of set tasks, or being positioned in repeatable postures, to measure change over time. Unfortunately, these scales have poor inter-rater reliability and are more useful if a single assessor is used.[34]

Associated reactions

Associated reactions are abnormal reflex movements which have been quantified as an indirect measure of spasticity.[35] This intention is conceptually inaccurate as spasticity and associated reactions are quite separate entities (see Chapter 3). In fact, the degree of associated reactions have shown poor correlation with isokinetic measurements of tone.[35] While another study did find a correlation between hypertonia (Ashworth Scale) and the degree of associated reaction (angle of elbow flexion during walking), it appeared that the correlation reflected the soft tissue component of the hypertonia more than the neural component;[36] more direct measurements of hypertonia are available. Associated reactions may be closely related to the patient's activity and effort,[35] and therefore might provide a non-specific and indirect measure of this effort. Again, there are probably more direct measurements available. A simple three point grading scale (mild, moderate or severe) is sometimes used in clinical practice, but there is no published literature on this. The use of associated reactions is therefore of limited value in the grading of spasticity.

Myometry

Spasticity in a muscle may reduce apparent strength of the antagonist muscle. This strength may be evaluated using a myometer. However, antagonist muscle strength may be affected by multiple factors in the UMN syndrome and, as such, this is not a useful measure of spasticity.

Performance and functional measurements

The Oswestry Scale of spasticity: control of voluntary movements

The Oswestry Scale illustrates the lack of understanding that commonly occurs when attempting to measure spasticity (Table 4.3). This scale is based on the common assumption that spasticity inter-

Table 4.3   The Oswestry Scale of spasticity grading: voluntary control of spastic limb[37]

0	**Solely spastic** No willed movement. Tonic reflexes or spinal reflexes present.
1	**Very severe spasticity** Movement very poor, being a total spastic synergy and in one pattern only, i.e. either only total extension if the limb is passively flexed or only total flexion from an extended position.
2	**Severe spasticity** Movement poor, being a marked total spastic synergy but in both flexion and extension patterns, i.e. the patient can flex the extended limb and extend the flexed limb, with or without some isolated proximal control.
3	**Moderate spasticity** Movement fair, spastic synergy, but some isolated control in a small range of movement at a distal joint (ankle or wrist).
4	**Mild spasticity** Movement good with isolated distal control possible in a good range, although spastic synergy is still apparent on reinforcement by resistance to the movement, or by effort exerted in another part of the body.
5	**No spasticity** Movement normal. No spastic synergy.

feres with the quality of movement.[37] However, spasticity may not be such a crucial factor in preventing voluntary movement (see Chapter 3).[38,39] Although other positive features of the UMN syndrome may interfere with function, it is the negative features which are the most disabling. Thus, functional impairment in the UMN syndrome is multifactorial and so functional measures should not be portrayed as measurements of spasticity. They may provide a 'useful parameter of activities of daily living' but do not reflect spasticity *per se*.[17]

In practice, the Scale seems sensitive to change in the acute setting but it has not yet been subjected to formal validity or reliability studies, despite being cited in a number of papers.[40] It closely resembles sections of the Fugel-Meyer motor assessment scale of the upper limb,[40] but is far easier to use.

SECTION THREE

CLINICAL TRIAL MEASUREMENTS

The clinical trial is a unique situation divorced from the reality of the every day clinical setting. Resources such as staff, time and equipment are available. In research, the clinician can attempt to improve upon the information yielded from the simple clinical tools. Some of the techniques frequently used in research as more or less direct measures of spasticity, such as electrogoniometry, isokinetic measurements and EMG, have already been mentioned. Computerised, three-dimensional gait analysis allows an indirect measure of spasticity by assessing one of its functional consequences — an abnormal gait. Pre-treatment assessment can confirm a visual analysis of gait or detect clinically inapparent abnormalities and can guide the clinician towards a treatment goal. However, the equipment is expensive and space and technical and interpretative skills are required. It is the gold standard of assessment of movement in gait and has been used in clinical trials of spasticity in cerebral palsy[41] but is not available to most clinicians.

CONCLUSION

Clinical measurement of spasticity is difficult. Clinical measurements of muscle tone cannot distinguish between the neural (spasticity) and biomechanical components. Those techniques available have not always been standardised or fully validated. Caution must be exerted when using instruments that evaluate the assumed consequences of spasticity, such as function. This chapter by no means covers all the options available. It is intended to highlight the variety of means available, their advantages and disadvantages, and to direct the reader to the literature on measurement of spasticity.

REFERENCES

1. Haas BM 1994 Measuring spasticity. A survey of current practice among health care professionals. Br J Ther Rehabil 2: 90–95
2. Katz RT, Rovai GP, Brait C, Rymer WZ 1992 Objective Quantification of Spastic Hypertonia: Correlation with Clinical Findings. Arch Phys Med Rehabil 73: 339–347
3. Struppler A 1985 Some new aspects of spasticity as revealed by clinical neurophysiology. In: Delwaide PJ, Young RR (eds) Clinical neurophysiology in Spasticity. Elsevier, Amsterdam, pp185–204
4. Young RR, Wiegner AW 1986 Spasticity. Clin Orthopaed 219: 51–62
5. Snow BJ, Tsui JKC, Bhatt MH, et al 1990 Treatment of spasticity with botulinum toxin: a double-blind study. Ann Neurol 28: 512–515
6. Campbell JW, Herbison GJ, Chen YT, Jaweed MM, Gussner CG 1991 Spontaneous electromyographic potentials in chronic spinal cord injured patients: relation to spasticity and length of nerve. Arch Phys Med Rehabil 72: 23–27
7. De Souza LH, Musa IM 1987 The measurement and assessment of spasticity. Clin Rehabil 1: 89–96
8. Dietz J, Berger W 1983 Normal and impaired regulation of muscle stiffness in gait. A new hypothesis about muscle hypotonia. Exper Neurol 79: 680

9. Hufschmidt A, Mauritz KH 1985 Chronic transformation of muscle in spasticity: a peripheral contribution to increased tone. J Neurol Neurosurg Psychiatry 48: 676–685

10. Ashworth B 1964 Preliminary trial of carisoprodol in multiple sclerosis. Practitioner 192: 540–542

11. Bohannon RW, Smith MB 1987 Inter-rater reliability of a modified Ashworth scale of muscle spasticity. Phys Ther 67: 206–207

12. Sloan RL, Sinclair E, Thompson S, Taylor S, Pentland E 1992 Interrater reliability of the modified Ashworth scale for spasticity in hemiplegic patients. Int J Rehabil Res 15: 158–161

13. Lee KC, Carson L, Kinnin E, Patterson V 1989 The Ashworth scale: a reliable and reproducible method of measuring spasticity. J Neurol Rehabil 3: 205–209

14. Haas BM, Bergstrom E, Jamous A, Bennie A 1996 The inter rater reliability of the original and of the modified Ashworth scale for the assessment of pasticity in patients with spinal cord injury. Spinal Cord 34: 560–564

15. Loubser PG, Narayan RK, Sandin KJ, Donovan WH, Russell RN 1991 Continuous infusion of intrathecal baclofen: Long-term effects on spasticity in spinal cord injury. Paraplegia 29: 48–64

16. Penn RD, Kroin JS 1985 Continuous intrathecal baclofen for severe spasticity. Lancet 7: 125–127

17. Katz RT, Rymer WZ 1989 Spastic hypertonia: mechanisms and measurement. Arch Phys Med Rehabil 70: 144–55

18. Carr JH, Shepherd RB, Nordholm L, Lynne D 1985 Investigation of a New Motor Assessment Scale for Stroke Patients. Phy Ther 65: 175–179

19. Borg TK, Caulfield JB 1980 Morphology of connective and endomysial connective tissues in skeletal muscle. Tissue Cell 13: 197–207

20. Mellin G, Olenius P, Setala H 1994 Comparison between three different inclinometers. Physiotherapy 80: 612–614

21. Watkins B, Darrah J, Pain K 1995 Reliability of passive ankle dorsiflexion measurements in children: Comparison of Universal and Biplane Goniometers. Paed Phys Ther 7: 3–8

22. Riddle DL, Rothstein JM, Lamb RL 1987 Goniometric reliability in a clinical setting: shoulder measurements. Phys Ther 67: 668–673

23. Low JL 1976 The reliability of joint measurement. Physiotherapy 62: 672–677

24. Ashton BB, Pickles B, Roll JW 1978 Reliability of goniometric measurements of hip motion in spastic cerebral palsy. Devel Med Child Neurol 20: 87–94

25. Norkin CC, White DJ 1995 Measurement of joint measurement. 2nd edition. A Guide to goniometry. FA Davies Company, Philadelphia

26. Bohannon RW, Lusardi MM 1991 Modified sphygmomanometer versus strain gauge hand held dynamometer. Arch Phys Med Rehabil 72: 911–914

27. Bajd T, Bowmand B 1982 Testing and modelling of spasticity. J Biomed Engineer 4: 90–96

28. Tardieu C, Colbeau-Justin, Lespargot A, et al 1976 An apparatus and a method for measuring the relationship of triceps surae torques to tibio-tarsal angles in Man. Eur J Applied Physiol 35: 11–20

29. Bohannon RW 1987 Variability and reliability of the pendulum test for spasticity using a Cybex isokinetic dynamometer. Phys Ther 67: 659–661

30. Seib TSP, Price R, Reyes MR, Lehmann JF 1994 The quantitative measurement of spasticity: Effect of cutaneous stimulation. Arch Phys Med Rehabil 75: 746–750

31. Malouin F, Boiteau M, Bonneau C, Pichard L, Bravo G 1989 Use of a hand held dynamometer for the evaluation of spasticity in a clinical setting. Physiother Canada 41: 126–134

32. Huskisson EC 1974 Measurement of pain. Lancet 9: 1127–1131

33. Downie WW, Leatham PA, Rhind VM, Pickup ME, Wright V 1978 The Visual Analogue Scale in the assessment of grip strength. Ann Rheum Dis 37: 382–384
34. Burry H 1972 Objective measurement of spasticity. Dev Med Child Neurol 14: 508–510
35. Dvir Z, Panturin E 1993 Measurement of spasticity and associated reactions in stroke patients before and after physiotherapeutic intervention. Clin Rehabil 7: 15–21
36. Dickstein R, Heffes Y, Abulaffio N 1996 Electromyographic and positional changes in the elbows of spastic hemiparetic patients during walking. Electroencephal Clin Neurophysiol 101: 491–496
37. Goff B 1976 Grading of spasticity and its effect on voluntary movement. Physiotherapy 62: 358–361
38. Rothwell J 1994 In: Control of human voluntary movement. 2nd edition. Chapman and Hall, London
39. Norton BJ, Bomze HA, Sahrmann SA, Eliasson SG, 1975 Correlation between gait speed and spasticity at the knee. Phys Ther 55: 355–359
40. Fugel-Meyer AR, Jaasko L, Leyman I, Olsson S, Steglind S 1975 The post stroke hemiplegic patient: A method for evaluation of physical performance. Scand J Rehabil Med 7: 13–31
41. Cosgrove AP, Corry IS, Graham HK 1994 Botulinum toxin in the management of the lower limb in cerebral palsy. Dev Med Child Neurol 36: 386–396

5. Spasticity rehabilitation: a rational approach to clinical management

Alan J. Thompson

INTRODUCTION

It is clear from the preceding chapters that spasticity is a complex entity which remains poorly understood and difficult to quantify. It is highly individual and variable, rarely occurs in isolation and it must never be managed as such. It is therefore hardly surprising that it poses major challenges in its management, which is often less than optimal. Spasticity will be dependent on a wide range of factors, most notable of which are the site of pathology, i.e. cerebral or spinal, and the pathological changes within the lesion. These may be more predictable following trauma of the spinal cord when compared to infectious or inflammatory pathologies. It must also be remembered that spasticity is a dynamic process that is movement dependent and therefore heavily and variably influenced by walking, transferring, etc. It is also strongly influenced by fatigue, temperature and stress and, similarly to the evaluation of blood pressure, a highly charged outpatient clinic is not necessarily the best place to evaluate spasticity.

Much of the difficulty in evaluating spasticity arises from the fact that it is frequently associated with other elements of the upper motor neurone (UMN) syndrome and therefore in the majority of clinical situations will be accompanied by other positive symptoms such as flexor and extensor spasms, clonus, and the more functionally disabling negative symptoms, notably weakness. Reducing spasticity may have a worsening effect on function by aggravating some of these symptoms, particularly weakness. It is not unusual, clinically, for patients to have severe flexor and extensor spasms but marked proximal weakness (involving the trunk and pelvis) with low postural tone. Even in a condition apparently as straightforward as hereditary spastic paraparesis where, at least in theory, reducing spasticity should improve mobility, there is not infrequently underlying weakness which becomes evident as the tone is reduced and this worsens mobility.

Over and above these complex interactions, spasticity frequently occurs in conditions, such as multiple sclerosis (MS), which produce a wide range of other symptoms, including cerebellar ataxia, sensory disturbance, sphincter dysfunction and severe fatigue. In such cases management of spasticity cannot be seen in isolation as attempts to influence it may potentially worsen other symptoms; many anti-spasticity medications tend to cause drowsiness and fatigue.

IMPACT OF SPASTICITY (TABLE 5.1)

Despite these complexities, it is possible to evaluate the impact of spasticity, although it is perhaps more clinically relevant to consider it together with the other features of the UMN syndrome, such as flexor and extensor spasms and pain. The major impact tends to focus on mobility, although effects on dexterity, the ability to manage bladder dysfunction and bulbar functions, such as respiration, swallowing and communication, should not be overlooked.

In relation to mobility, the most profound effect is on gait. Spasticity tends to slow mobility, making walking more laborious and effortful and resulting in a progressive reduction in exercise tolerance. There is an increasing tendency to a more laboured gait pattern, with an increased risk of falling, as a consequence. Increasing spasticity and worsening posture frequently result in, or accentuate pain in the lumbar area. However, mobility covers a much broader

Table 5.1 Impact of spasticity

Mobility	Gait
	Transfers
	bed to chair
	toilet
	car
Dexterity	Bed mobility
	Feeding
	Writing
	Personal care
Bladder management	
Bulbar function	Swallowing
	Respiration
	Communication

area, particularly when considering more disabled patients. Transfers including chair to bed, toilet or car may be severely compromised, and bed mobility may become extremely difficult if not impossible. Spasms may also make gait unsafe and cause problems with transfers resulting in falls and, in more severely disabled patients, great difficulties for carers.

Spasticity may also result in a loss of dexterity which has a direct impact on the patient's ability to attend to their own personal care and feeding, and may also make writing more difficult. In patients who are paraplegic, upper limb spasticity may restrict transfers and, if very severe, limit the ability to use a wheelchair. In patients with bladder dysfunction, spasticity may also interfere with the ability to carry out clean intermittent self-catheterisation (CISC), both because of the reduction in upper limb function and increased lower limb adductor tone.

Rarely, spasticity may compromise bulbar function. Truncal spasticity may affect respiration and swallowing and, in some patients with cerebral palsy, communication may be a major problem.

In summary, spasticity, with or without other positive phenomena of the UMN syndrome, may have a major impact on a wide range of key functions of daily living and, therefore by definition, worsen disability and increase handicap. Spasticity may also cause considerable pain as a result of a number of different processes — pain associated with flexor and extensor spasms, chronic lumbar pain as a result of poor posture and increased tone, and the deep gnawing pain which is frequently present in a hypertonic limb. This symptom can often predominate in the more disabled patient and has a profound effect on their quality of life.

AN APPROACH TO MANAGEMENT

Given the complexities outlined above and in previous chapters it is clear that a practical and somewhat pragmatic approach to the management of spasticity is necessary. The first and most important point is that one is not managing spasticity itself but the person with spasticity. Indeed, one may go further and state that the removal of spasticity may in itself be detrimental as it is not infrequently used by patients as a crutch on which to stand and walk. Thus, the removal of spasticity *per se* is not a treatment goal. Each patient presents a different and unique pattern of neurological dysfunction which must be addressed. Ideally the main aim of intervention is to improve the level of function. This is particularly the case in patients who are not severely disabled. Appropriate intervention should result in improvements in all aspects of health status including disability, handicap and health-related quality of life. The second treatment aim should be to remove pain resulting either from spasticity itself or from associated flexor and extensor spasms. Such pain is frequently very disabling and therefore its management will also result in improvements in disability and quality of life. Intervention must also be aimed at preventing the complications of spasticity, such as contractures and pressure sores, benefits which will not be appreciated unless they are not achieved! Finally, in patients with very severe disability, treatment of spasticity may be initiated to ease care. This should improve quality of life of the patient and that of their carers.

MANAGEMENT STRATEGY (Fig. 5.1)

The first step in any management strategy is to identify which of the aims outlined above can be achieved. In other words, is the spasticity impairing function, causing pain, likely to lead to complications,

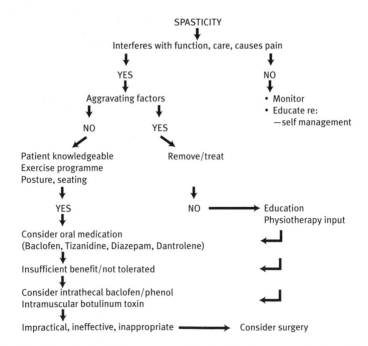

Fig. 5.1   A flowchart outlining an approach to the clinical management of spasticity.

or is it interfering with care? If not, then it may well be that no direct action needs to take place. However, even at this early stage patient education is crucial. Self-management is the cornerstone of a successful strategy in this as with many other neurological symptoms. If a patient has a better understanding of the nature of spasticity, the importance of good posture, stretching, standing and adopting patterns of movement which discourage increasing spasticity, then they will have much better control of this symptom and a clearer idea of when to seek help. Much more attention needs to be given to providing an education programme which is best carried out by a physiotherapist, although this is not absolutely essential.

The second step in management strategy is identification of any factors which may aggravate spasticity (Table 5.2). This is relevant at all stages of severity of spasticity but is most appropriate in the more disabled patient where many of these factors may coexist. Their detection may be hampered by the patient's lack of awareness, either as a result of severe sensory disturbance or cognitive dysfunction. Patients with spasticity frequently have bladder dysfunction with incomplete emptying which will predispose to urinary tract infections (UTIs). Bowel dysfunction, producing constipation and impaction, is also a common symptom often unrecognised in severely disabled, bed-bound patients. Ironically it is occasionally the orthotic devices provided for the patient with spasticity and weakness which may on the one hand support the limb but on the other increase spasticity if they are ill-fitting or too tight. Lengthy lists of aggravating factors are often cited but are still often overlooked with clinicians increasing anti-spasticity medication to patients with infected bed-sores, etc.

The physiotherapist is the other key player in the treatment of spasticity and in many instances is not involved in management at an early enough stage. The role of the physiotherapist is not just to

---

Table 5.2   Spasticity: aggravating factors

- Urinary tract infections (UTIs)
- Bowel impaction
- Skin irritation/ulceration
- Ingrown toe nails
- Increased sensory stimuli from
  — tight-fitting clothes or orthoses
- Deep venous thrombosis (DVT)
- Undetected fracture

treat spasticity, but also to define problems and help to prepare the management plan. If, however, spasticity continues to interfere with dysfunction despite this expert input then it may be necessary to consider medication. This should always be given in association with, and monitored by, the physiotherapist, particularly if the delicate balance between negative and positive symptoms is to be managed appropriately. Many medical practitioners have given anti-spasticity medication independently of the physiotherapist, often in high doses, and indeed without physiotherapy intervention, which in turn aggravates the underlying or associated weakness. It is therefore not surprising that many patients are very wary of anti-spasticity agents and are very reluctant to use them.

If a single oral medication is insufficient, it may be necessary to combine medications which act at different sites, i.e. baclofen and dantrolene or baclofen and tizanidine. Such combinations also increase the side-effect profile but may on occasion be well tolerated. If a combination is unsuccessful then it may be necessary to consider a more invasive management such as the intrathecal administration of baclofen or phenol or the intramuscular administration of botulinum toxin (BTX) or nerve blocks. There are, however, occasions when focal treatment with either BTX or phenol nerve block may be more appropriate than oral medication, e.g. in an unconscious patient with dystonic posturing of one or both feet. Surgical intervention may be particularly useful in the correction of joint deformities but is rarely required to treat spasticity *per se*.

6. Evaluation of interventions in the management of spasticity: treatment goals and outcome measures

Davina Richardson

INTRODUCTION

In general terms, neurological rehabilitation aims to maximise functional potential and minimise secondary complications, ultimately to improve quality of life. The two aims are not mutually exclusive and their emphasis may change depending on the level of disability of the patient.

Spasticity is one symptom of central nervous system (CNS) damage that is responsive to treatment and thus it receives more attention than the other features of the upper motor neurone (UMN) syndrome. The first step in the treatment of spasticity is to identify the clinical problems that it creates. The question of why we want to treat spasticity must be carefully considered.[1] A reduction of spasticity may not improve function and in some cases may actually reduce function further.[2] Secondly, a treatment goal must be specified together with a means of evaluating its achievement. Without these it is impossible to determine the effectiveness of a treatment. The third step is to choose the most effective means (treatment) of achieving the goal.

This chapter describes the initial stages of this decision-making process; specific treatment issues will be discussed in later chapters. Section one presents a model of goal setting and section two discusses the selection of outcome measures appropriate to the identified treatment goals.

SECTION ONE

SETTING TREATMENT GOALS

Simply aiming to reduce spasticity is not a final treatment goal; there must be a purpose behind it. A clinical problem, or sequence of problems, arising in the patient as a consequence of spasticity must be identified; these have been discussed in previous chapters. Having decided that anti-spasticity therapy is indicated, treatment goals can be set.

A MODEL OF GOAL SETTING IN THE MANAGEMENT OF SPASTICITY IN REHABILITATION

The process of goal setting starts with a thorough understanding of the pathophysiology of the clinical problem. The treatment process designed to achieve the final goal of therapy can usually be divided into a series of steps based upon a sequence of pathophysiological events underlying the clinical problem (Fig. 6.1). Each step is a short-term goal to be achieved on the way to achieving longer-term goals and can be evaluated by its own specific outcome measure. They thus provide precision of treatment and a way of monitoring progress towards the long-term goal. Failure to achieve the long-term goal may be traced back to failure to adequately achieve some of the short-term goals. Conversely, failure to achieve the long-term goal despite success at the earlier levels may bring to light an incorrect assumption — for example, that reduction in spasticity would improve function.

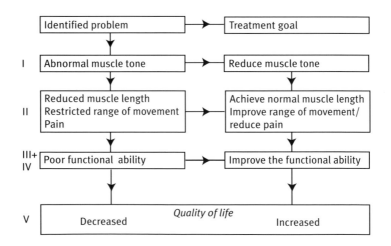

Fig. 6.1   A five level model of goal setting.

LEVELS OF TREATMENT GOALS

In this section, a model of goal setting using a step ladder approach will be outlined followed by an example of its application to a clinical problem. It should be emphasised that this is a model of rehabilitation of spasticity and not a general model of rehabilitation.

Level one

The level one treatment goal is an attack on the basic pathophysiological mechanism assumed to be the root of the identified clinical problem. The goal is usually a reduction in elevated muscle tone (e.g. spasticity). Depending upon the specific situation, therapy may need to be directed at the neural or biomechanical components of the hypertonia or both (see later treatment chapters). Reducing the muscle tone allows progression to the second level.

Level two

There are two fundamental treatment goals at this level — achieving normal muscle length and a pain-free full range of joint motion. Clearly, both require a reduction in muscle tone (level one). Failure to achieve these two goals will severely hamper any attempts to gain function (level four). They are also necessary to avoid contracture and deformity, which may by themselves be treatment goals.

Level three

By reducing tone (level one) and increasing muscle length and passive range of movement (level two), the area of assisted functional tasks of daily living can be addressed. These may be regarded as passive functional tasks, done for, rather than by, the patient. Clinical problems in this realm include:

1. Difficulty washing a body part (e.g. gaining access to the palm with tightly flexed fingers)
2. Difficulty dressing a body part (e.g. getting an arm into a sleeve)
3. Difficulty positioning body (e.g. sitting, standing, lying). These clinical problems form the treatment goals.

A wide variety of treatments are available to achieve goals at levels one to three. Because of this and the diversity of the impact of spasticity, goal setting at levels two and three requires the use of targets related to the individual patient and specific intervention. For example, if splinting is necessary to maintain muscle length then tolerance of splints can be a short-term goal. Similarly, if regular stretches are required, the ability of the patient to be able to effectively stretch their own affected muscle can be an important sub-goal.

Level four

Level four goals involve active movement of the affected limb that leads to the independent performance of functional tasks. Treatment goals at level four always depend upon:

1. Antagonistic and agonist control/strength
2. Reciprocal activity in muscles
3. Active voluntary movement and control at a joint or in a limb
4. Functional tasks.

Functional goals are usually quite specific. Thus, within a global level four goal of improved hand function, specific functional tasks such as handshaking, gripping a cup and writing, would be identified. Failure at levels one to three make it unlikely that the level four goal would be achieved. Conversely, success at this level depends upon the assumption being correct that the basic (level one) problem (e.g. spasticity) is contributing substantially to the dysfunction. Success at levels one to three will not lead to success at level four (functional gain) if this assumption is incorrect. The point has been made many times that spasticity is frequently not the principal cause of functional impairment in the UMN syndrome. Other negative components, such as weakness and loss of distal dexterity, will strongly influence functional goals, as will associated cognitive and sensory impairments. The skill of the clinician is to determine the influence of each of the different factors and how they combine to create the problem.

Level five

The ultimate goal in rehabilitation is a reduction in handling and an improved quality of life for the individual. In practice, most treatments aim at achieving level four, with the assumption (or hope) that improved quality of life (level five) will follow.

THE WHO CLASSIFICATION OF THE CONSEQUENCES OF ILLNESS

The World Health Organisation (WHO) classification of three types of consequences of illness — impairment, disability and handicap (Table 6.1) — has been endorsed.[3] Impairment relates to the clinical signs. This would include any of the positive or negative phenomena of the UMN syndrome (Table 1.1), including spasticity, as well as the secondary complications of pain, and soft tissue and joint changes. Disability describes abnormal performance of the individual which, in the UMN syndrome, usually results not just from spasticity but from the combined effects of the whole syndrome. Finally, inability to walk due to spasticity may present a handicap, by preventing the patient from going to work.

It is clinically useful to approach management with this classification in mind. In relation to the model of goal setting presented earlier in this chapter, impairment broadly corresponds with levels one and two, disability with levels three and four, and handicap with level five.

USING THE MODEL

Consider a subject with increased tone (spasticity) in the fingers leading to flexed posturing of the hand. The treatment goal may be to improve hand function so that the patient is able to open the hand to grasp an object. In order to achieve this treatment goal, we must reduce tone in the finger flexors (level one), then increase muscle length of the finger flexors and range of motion of the joints, ideally without causing pain (level two). In achieving the first two levels, the patient is able to work with the hand to increase strength and voluntary control of the finger flexors and extensors in order to improve hand function (level four). It is likely that an improved quality of life (level five) will follow.

Table 6.1   WHO classification of disease consequences

Impairment	Any loss or abnormality of psychological, physiological or anatomical structure or function
Disability	Any restriction or lack of ability to perform an activity in a manner or within the range considered normal
Handicap	The way in which an impairment or disability influences the individual's ability to fulfil a role that is normal for that individual

GENERAL GOAL SETTING INFORMATION

Treatment goals may be of two types – patient related or therapy related. Although they may be the same goals, they may also be very different. Goals of each type may be set simultaneously. Treatment goals must be specific to the individual, prioritised and, most of all, realistic. This demands adequate discussion with the patient, or with their carers if the patients are incapable. All parties concerned with the treatment of the individual should be aware of the goal set, even if they are not directly related to its achievement. It is advisable to set only one treatment goal at a time; this focuses attention and increases the likelihood of success. Having set the treatment goals, ways by which to measure the success in achieving these goals must be chosen.

SECTION TWO

OUTCOME MEASUREMENT

Measurement of health-related outcomes are important to evaluate the effect and efficacy of therapeutic intervention.[4] Careful outcome measurement allows prediction of those patients who will benefit most from treatment, identification of the most appropriate intervention and ensures realistic expectations from that treatment. Most importantly, it should lead to improved patient management. This section will outline the principles of outcome measurement and provide a practical guide to the selection of a measurement tool.

GENERAL PRINCIPLES OF OUTCOME MEASUREMENT

For the clinician to make the best use of an outcome measure, the question to be answered and the purpose of the measurement must be clear. There are a large number of outcome measures available,[5] and these must be evaluated in terms of both clinical utility and scientific validity.[4] To be clinically useful, an outcome measure must be simple to use, accessible, easily communicated, acceptable to the patient, brief to apply and provide the information required. A measurement tool should also be scientifically sound, with three properties:

1. **Reliability** — are the results from the measure accurate, consistent, reliable over time and reproducible?
2. **Validity** — does it measure what it purports to measure?
3. **Responsiveness** — does the measure detect clinically important change?

These properties are not, 'all or nothing' concepts;[6] each measurement tool can be judged on the strength of each property. For example, goniometric measurement of a joint angle may have strong validity but poor reliability. The clinician should be aware that very few of the many instruments available for measuring neurological outcome have undergone rigorous evaluation of these three properties. This problem can be partially alleviated by using a number of measurements in any one instance, combining perhaps one strongly valid measure with a strongly reliable measure. Care should also be taken when using measurement tools borrowed from other medical specialities (e.g. rheumatology), as there will be no normative data for their use in neurology. However, such measures may provide useful serial data.

SOME CLINICAL OUTCOME MEASURES

Table 6.2 lists some of the many outcome measures available that the author has found clinically useful in the management of spasticity. The reader must be aware that not all the tests listed have been subject to scientific evaluation in terms of validity, reliability and responsiveness.

The limitations of some of the outcome measures relating to spasticity (e.g. Ashworth Scale) were discussed previously in Chapter 4. Figs. 6.2–6.5 present diagrammatically how some of these measures fit in with the step model of goal setting presented earlier. At certain treatment steps there may be no validated measurement tools for the specific goal, especially where these are highly individualised, such as hand hygiene and writing tasks. In these cases, the clinician usually resorts to visual analogue scales or other forms of subjective rating scales. Transition questions have also found popularity for this situation.[7]

SUBJECTIVE ASSESSMENT OF THE TREATMENT

Transition questions

Transition questions have been used in rheumatology and make use of subjective data.[8] They question the patient on the outcome of a treatment and are related to the specific goal that was set initially. For example, if the treatment goal was to be able to get a jacket on more easily, the question might be, 'Has the task of putting your jacket on and off changed since you received treatment?' A simple seven point scoring system is used (Table 6.3). Thus, the transition question varies and is specific to the goal but the response scale is the same.

Table 6.2   A selection of outcome measures

Impairment (level one)	Outcome measure	Focal disability (levels two & three	Outcome measure
Muscle tone (resistance to passive movement)	Ashworth Scale[11]	Walking speed	Timed 10 metre walk[19] 6 minute walking test[20]
Pain	Visual analogue scale[12]	Standing balance	Berg balance scale[21]
Range of movement	Universal goniometer[13] Electrogoniometer[14]	Manual dexterity	Nine-hole peg test[22] Jebsen hand function test[23] Rivermead motor upper limb[18]
Muscle strength	Jamar grip meter[15] Myometry[16]		
Movement	Motricity index[17] Rivermead motor assessment scale[18]		
Functional disability (level four)	**Outcome measure**	**Handicap Quality of life (level five)**	**Outcome measure**
Activities of daily living	Barthel Index[24] Functional independence measure[25] Nottingham 10 point ADL index	Handicap	Nottingham Health Profile[27] Short form 36 questionnaire[28]

CHOOSING THE RIGHT OUTCOME MEASURE

In the management of spasticity more mistakes are made when choosing the treatment goal than when deciding upon appropriate outcome measurements of that goal. For example, it may be assumed, incorrectly for a particular patient, that reducing tone will enable them to move better and improve function. A functional outcome measure is appropriate for the goal, but the goal is unrealistic.

It may be helpful when choosing an outcome measure to consider it in terms of the clinical problem that it is evaluating. Thus, for the WHO classification, there are measures of impairment (muscle tone – Ashworth Scale), disability (hand function – nine-hole peg test) and handicap (a quality of life measure). Similarly, outcome measures may need to meet a purpose beyond simple measurement. Those which

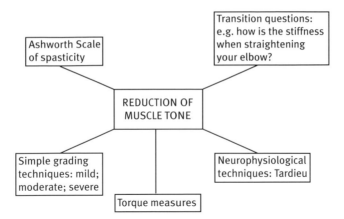

Fig. 6.2 Examples of outcome measures for level one goal setting: reduction of tone.

measure activities of daily living (ADL), are considered 'predictive'[9] as they are good predictors of community placement of an individual.[10]

Bearing all this in mind, it is probably most helpful to reiterate an earlier discussion and interrogate specific outcome measures in the following way.[5]

● Is it actually relevant?
● Is it a valid measure of what you wish to assess?
● What is its reliability?
● Is it sensitive enough to detect the change/difference expected?
● Is it simple enough to be used in the clinical setting?
● Can the results be communicated easily to others?
● Is there a better measure available?

Attention to these questions will help decide the best outcome measure.

Table 6.3 Scoring a transition question

BETTER	much better	7
	moderately better	6
	slightly better	5
THE SAME	no change	4
WORSE	slightly worse	3
	moderately worse	2
	much worse	1

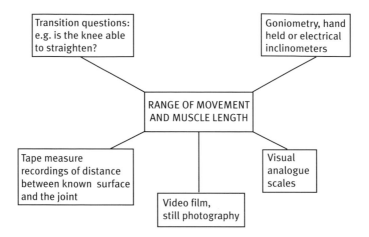

Fig. 6.3 Examples of outcome measures for level two goal setting: range of movement and muscle length.

WHEN TO APPLY AN OUTCOME MEASURE

All rehabilitation intervention is based on decisions made after a detailed assessment of the individual's situation. Measurement at the time of initial assessment, before starting treatment, is essential. Ideally, a series of baseline measures should be taken over a period of time to identify the rate of change that may be occurring.

The timing of subsequent measures, after beginning treatment, depends upon the expected time course of the corresponding treatment goal. These may vary widely, especially between treatment goal levels. For example, botulinum toxin injections may produce maximal weakening of spastic muscles after a week (level one) but the splinting that this allows might not fully reduce the accompanying biomechanical contribution to tone and increase range of movement for several more weeks (level two). Subsequent improvement in hand function (levels three and four) may take even longer, especially if strengthening of muscles and relearning are required. Outcome measures may therefore need to be administered at different times in order to detect change. Past experience might allow the clinician to predict when change will occur and match the timing of the measures appropriately.

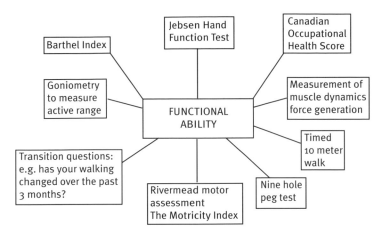

Fig. 6.4 Examples of outcome measures for levels three and four goal setting: functional ability.

CONCLUSION

The clinician is faced with a large volume of information relating to the setting of treatment goals and selection of outcome measures. The important points to remember in the clinic are simplicity and ease of application. Keep the treatment goals specific and realistic, and the measurements relevant. Be clear on the information that you want. Time spent setting the treatment goal and choosing the appropriate outcome measure will be time well spent.

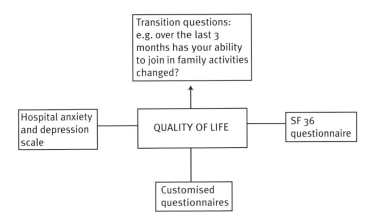

Fig. 6.5 Examples of outcome measures for level five goal setting: quality of life.

REFERENCES

1. Landau WM 1974 Spasticity: the fable of a neurological demon and the emperor's new therapy. Ann Neurol 31: 217–219
2. Ochs G, Stuppler A, Meyerson BA, et al 1989 Intrathecal baclofen for long-term treatment of spasticity: a multi-centre study. J Neurol Neurosurg Psychiatry 52: 933–939
3. Duckworth D 1984 The need for a standard terminology and classification of disablement. In: Granger CV, Gresham GE (eds) Functional Assessment in Rehabilitation Medicine. Williams and Wilkins, Baltimore, pp 1–13
4. Hobart JC 1996 Evaluating neurological outcome measures: bare essentials. J Neurol Neurosurg Psychiatry 60: 127–130
5. Wade D 1992 In: Measurement in Neurological Rehabilitation, Oxford University Press
6. Rothstein JM 1985 Measurement and clinical practice: theory and application. In: Rothstein JM (ed) Measurement in Physical Therapy. Churchill Livingstone, London, pp 1–47
7. Fitzpatrick R, Ziebland S, Jenkinson C, Mowat A, Mowat A 1993 Transition questions to assess outcomes in rheumatoid arthritis. Br J Rheumatol 32: 807–811
8. Mahoney FL, Barthel DW 1965 Functional evaluation: the Barthel Index. Maryland State Med J 14: 61–65
9. Jeffry LIH 1993 Aspects of selecting outcome measures to demonstrate the effectiveness of comprehensive rehabilitation. Br J Occup Ther 5: 394–400
10. Fricke J 1993 Measuring Outcomes in Rehabilitation: A Review. Br J Occup Ther 56: 217–221
11. Ashworth B 1964 Preliminary trial of carisoprodol in multiple sclerosis. Practitioner 192: 540–542
12. Huskisson EC 1974 Measurement of pain. Lancet 9: 1127–1131
13. Norkin CC, White DJ 1975 Measurement of Joint Motion. A Guide to Goniometry. Philadelphia, FA Davies
14. Nicol AC 1987 A new flexible electrogoniometer with widespread applications. In: Jonson B (ed) International series on Biomechanics: Biomechanics X-B. Human Kinetics Publications, Champaign, Illinois, pp 1029–1033
15. Mathiowetz V, Weber K, Volland G, Kashman N 1984 Reliability and validity of grip and pinch strength evaluations. J Hand Surg Am 92: 222–226
16. Wiles CM, Karni Y, Nicklin J 1990 Laboratory testing of muscle function in the management of neuromuscular disease. J Neurol Neurosurg Psychiatry 53: 384–387
17. Demeurisse G, Demol O, Robaye E 1980 Motor evaluation in vascular hemiplegia. Eur Neurol 19: 382–389
18. Lincoln NB, Leadbetter D 1979 Assessment of motor function in stroke patients. Physiotherapy 65: 48–51
19. Bradstater ME, De Bruin H, Gowland C, Clarke BM 1983 Hemiplegic gait: analysis of temporal variables. Arch Phys Med Rehabil 64: 583–587
20. Lipkin DP, Scriven AJ, Crake T, Poole-Wilson PA 1986 Six minute walking test for assessing exercise capacity in chronic heart failure. Br Med J 292: 653–655
21. Berg K, Wood-Dauphinee S, Williams JI, Maki B 1992 Measuring balance in the elderly: validation of an instrument. Can J Public Health (July/August supplement) 2: 57–11
22. Mathiowetz V, Weber K, Kashman N, Weber K 1985 Adult norms for the nine-hole peg test of finger dexterity. Occup Ther J Res 5: 24–37
23. Jebsen RH, Trieschmann R, Trotter N, Howard LA 1969 An objective and standardised test of hand function. Arch Phys Rehabil 50: 311–319

24. Collin C, Wade D, Davis S, Horne B 1988 The Barthel ADL index: a reliability study. International Disability Studies 10: 61–63
25. Granger CV, Hamilton BB, Sherwin FS 1986 Guide for the use of the uniform data set for medical rehabilitation. Uniform Data System for Medical Rehabilitation Project Office, Buffalo General Hospital, New York
26. Ebrahim S, Nouri F, Barer D 1985 Measuring disability after stroke. J Epidemiol Comm Health 39: 86–89
27. Hunt SM, Mckenna SP McEwan J 1980 A quantitative approach to perceived health status: a validation study. J Epidemiol Comm Health 34: 281–286
28. Ware JE 1993 SF-36 Health Survey. Manual and Interpretation Guide. The Health Institute, New England Medical Center, Boston, Massachusetts

7. Physiotherapy management of established spasticity

Susan Edwards

INTRODUCTION

Increased tone is a common manifestation of neurological pathology and is often a key determinant of the severity of disability. The primary aim of physiotherapy is to enable the restoration of optimal function. However, the variety of therapeutic approaches differ significantly in the analysis and interpretation of the diagnostic term so frequently used — 'spasticity'. The classical definition of spasticity is that it is 'a motor disorder characterised by a velocity-dependent increase in tonic stretch reflexes with exaggerated tendon jerks resulting from hyperexcitability of the stretch reflex'.[1] While this may be an accurate definition of one of the 'neural' components of hypertonia (see Chapter 3),[2] it is of little relevance to the patient or the therapist. The biomechanical components of hypertonia (reduced muscle and tendon compliance) and the negative features of weakness and loss of dexterity[3,4] may be of greater significance to the patient. Indeed O'Dwyer and colleagues[3] concluded that 'while hypertonia remains an important problem following cerebral lesions, it would appear that the amount of attention directed to reflex hyperexcitability is out of proportion to its effects'. As has already been stated in earlier chapters, the other positive features of the upper motor neurone (UMN) syndrome are also commonly referred to as spasticity, despite being clearly distinct clinically and pathophysiologically. Even the increased tone seen in the immediate aftermath of head injury is labelled spasticity. All this lack of clarity in terminology leads to confusion, particularly when discussing therapeutic strategies.

Physiotherapy treatment approaches differ in their emphasis with regard to the management of tone and the prevention of biomechanical changes in muscles. For example, Bobath[5] advocates the control of abnormal reflex activity and the underlying tone to improve co-ordination of movement. In contrast, Carr et al[2] advocates direct movement training towards improving performance of everyday actions thereby enabling the patient to learn control of muscle activity and develop strength and endurance during functional motor performance.

It would seem that advocates of the different treatment approaches are moving closer together in that all recognise that abnormal tone and biomechanical changes in muscle are integrally linked in the management of patients with spasticity. Specific inhibitory mobilisation of affected muscle groups is now advocated as a key component of the treatment of patients with increased tone by the British Adult Bobath Tutors Association but, unfortunately, there is no current literature to support this change of emphasis.

This chapter will begin with an analysis of the key features of normal movement, illustrating how these becomes disordered in spasticity and the UMN syndrome and the implications that this has for physiotherapy. The second section will describe specific physiotherapeutic measures employed in the rehabilitation of spasticity.

AN ANALYSIS OF NORMAL MOVEMENT

Analysis of movement may be considered in the context of five key determinants:

- Postural tone
- Reciprocal innervation
- Sensory motor feedback and feedforward
- Balance reactions
- Biomechanical properties of muscle.

Postural tone

The usual clinical definition of muscle tone is the resistance to passive movement when the patient is in a state of voluntary relaxation.[8] However, therapists also view tone in a broader, postural context as 'the state of readiness of the body musculature in preparation for the maintenance of a posture or the performance of a movement'.[9] Normal postural tone is infinitely variable according to postural and environmental demands. It enables an individual to maintain an upright posture against the force of gravity whilst at the same time allowing selective movement for functional tasks.

Clinical implications

The therapeutic management of patients with increased tone is determined by its severity and distribution. The base of support is of particular significance, this being described as the area within the boundaries of each point of contact with the supporting surface.[10] A large and supportive base of support is conducive to relaxation and a general lowering of postural tone. Conversely, an unstable, narrow base of support produces a heightening of postural tone. One has only to compare responses when lying on a comfortable bed to standing on a grassy verge on the edge of a precipice to appreciate the difference.

The choice of position when treating patients with spasticity is therefore of tremendous importance. It might be assumed that lying would be the position of choice. However, spastic hypertonia tends to dominate in stereotypical patterns which may be exacerbated when the patient is lying down. Such patients may need modification of the supporting surface in order for them to accommodate to it. Positioning in bed, passive/ active movements, posture in the wheelchair and standing will all be influenced by the underlying tone. Equally, the manner in which these activities are carried out will in turn influence the prevailing tone.

Reciprocal innervation

This is a term used by therapists to describe the graded interaction of agonists, antagonists and synergists during the maintenance of a posture or the performance of a movement.[5] Movement may require contraction of the antagonist at the same time as the agonist muscle (co-contraction), a process which is controlled in part by varying the amount of reciprocal inhibition which exists normally between agonist and antagonist: when co-contraction is required, reciprocal inhibition is suppressed and when unopposed agonist contraction is needed, reciprocal inhibition is facilitated. Dynamic co-contraction describes the graded interaction of agonist and antagonist to provide controlled movement and postural stability as the task at hand requires. Conversely, static co-contraction refers to a pathological state, as in dystonia and the UMN syndrome, whereby failure of normal reciprocal inhibition results in inappropriate co-contraction which inhibits normal modulation and restricts movement and thereby function (Chapter 3). However, some therapists consider reciprocal inhibition to be an abnormal process, which is at odds with the physiological literature which describes reciprocal inhibition as a normal phenomenon and a component of reciprocal innervation. Although inappropriate reciprocal inhibition in the UMN syndrome can lead to underactivity of muscles, as explained in Chapter 3, this is through disordered *control* of a normal phenomenon. As with spasticity, this lack of clarity and consistency in the use of terminology can lead to confusion.

Reciprocal innervation is essential for balance, in maintaining the centre of gravity within the base of support and in providing body stability through postural adjustments which occur prior to and during the performance of a movement.[11]

Clinical implications

A common feature of spasticity is an associated increase in the degree of antagonistic muscle contraction seen during alternating muscle actions.[12] Dominance of certain muscles produces the state of static co-contraction described above, as opposed to the dynamic stability characteristic of normal postural control.[10] This state has also been referred to as 'spastic dystonia' (see Chapter 2).

This imbalance of muscle activity clearly has implications for balance and for the sequence of postural adjustments which occur prior to and during the performance of movement. These are influenced by the support provided to an individual and by the speed at which the movement is performed.[13,14] Therefore, therapists should give consideration to the use of standing aids and the speed at which the patient is able to move. For example, the use of a tilt table, where the patient is fully supported and rarely stands in a fully upright position, will alter the recruitment order of these adjustments. Also, the inability to move as quickly as normal subjects means that postural adjustments will be made more slowly.

Sensory motor feedback and feed forward system

The production of voluntary movement has been described as sequential, consisting of the idea or reason to move — the motor plan — which is constantly updated to fit the requirements of the muscles involved in the movement, and the execution of the movement.[15]

Postures and movements are said to be guided by a mixture of motor programmes which can be viewed as a set of commands that are capable of carrying out movement without the use of feedback.[16] Providing one is able to move in a normal way, constantly utilising a wide variety of motor programmes, these will continue to be reinforced and refined by repetition.[10] Adjustments can be made as the need arises but for the production of a functional movement, such as writing, it is argued that there must be a common set of instructions.[17]

Motor learning is associated with practice or experience leading to relatively permanent changes in the capability for skilled performance.[18] It is therefore an active process, dependent upon the continual interaction between neural and musculoskeletal structures.

Clinical implications

The established patterns of spasticity and the underlying weakness create new motor programmes that are dictated by the stereotyped activity. The resultant effort and compensatory strategies which are adopted to counteract the dominant spastic posturing and the underlying weakness produce an abnormal sensory input to the CNS.[19]

Any impairment in the neural control of movement and/or changes in the musculoskeletal system will affect the quality of performance. The aim of physiotherapy is to modify this stereotypical response by facilitation of more normal movement patterns. Prolonged use of a limited repertoire of movement patterns creates a dominant abnormal response which becomes increasingly difficult to reverse. Once established, re-education of more purposeful movement can sometimes only be achieved with outside intervention such as localised injections of botulinum toxin (BTX) to weaken the dominant spastic muscles.[20]

Balance reactions

Postural control provides stability and orientation and requires:

• The integration of sensory information to assess the position and motion of the body in space
• The ability to generate forces for controlling body position.[21]

Postural adjustments occur continually to maintain the centre of gravity within the base of support. Any alteration in the location of the centre of gravity necessitates continuous postural adjustments and even the smallest movement has to be countered by modification of postural tone throughout the body musculature.[5]

Shumway-Cook and Wollacott[21] describe balance reactions in terms of the ankle, hip and stepping strategies. For example, the postural sway in standing occurs with movement primarily at the ankles, the rest of the body remaining upright. If greater demands are placed upon the balance mechanism or larger, faster movements are required, the discrete movement at the ankle may prove inadequate and movement at the hips becomes more pronounced. Finally, if all else fails and the centre of gravity is displaced outside the base of support, balance is hopefully restored by a stepping response in the direction to which balance is displaced.

Clinical implications

Normal reciprocal innervation and a full range of movement at the joint around which the movement occurs are essential for effective balance. Both are commonly impaired in extensor spasticity of the lower limb. A typical example is the positive support reaction whereby the foot is unable to adapt to and accept the base of support (see also Chapter 2). The patient is unable to transfer their weight over the full surface of the foot and the ankle remains in a degree of plantarflexion. The compensatory response is flexion at the hip to maintain the body weight over the supporting surface.

It is also important to remember that patients with impaired movement control are often apprehensive, realising that their response to sudden and unexpected events may be inadequate to maintain balance. Movements are consequently slower and the background postural tone higher, particularly in standing and walking, in anticipation of potential falls.[20]

Biomechanical properties of muscle

In the UMN syndrome, changes occur to both the intrinsic muscle structure and to external structures such as connective tissue which leads to muscle stiffness and contracture.

Skeletal muscle fibres are of three types, slow oxidative (SO), fast gylcolytic (FG) and fast oxidative glycolytic (FOG). Muscles with predominantly SO fibres participate in longer lasting but relatively weak contractions, such as in postural control, whereas those with predominantly FG fibres generate large forces but are more readily fatigued. Motor units are recruited according to the size principal[22] and are in the order of SO, FOG, FG.

Muscles alter their characteristics in response to function and activity.[4] In the UMN syndrome, the changes which occur in the biomechanical properties of muscle may be considered in terms of:

- Neural control, whereby the sustained activity of hypertonic muscles produces a change in fibre type from FG to SO[6]
- The postural effects of neurological impairment, whereby immobility leads to atrophy which is more pronounced in SO than FG[23,24]
- Alteration in the muscle structure itself with remodelling of the intramuscular connective tissue and a reduction in the number of sarcomeres in those muscles held in a shortened position leading to increased muscle stiffness and contracture.[23]

Hufschmidt and Mauritz[25] postulate that 'elastic and velocity-independent plastic resistance are enhanced in long standing spasticity' and support the hypothesis of secondary changes in muscle as an additional component of increased tone. Additionally, even with the sustained muscle contraction associated with hypertonia, there is rarely hypertrophy and more often atrophy. This may be due to the inability of the individual to move through a full range of movement.

Clinical implications

It is possible that a change in the dominant biomechanical property of muscle from FG to SO, brought about by continuous activity in hypertonia and immobility, might affect the normal recruitment order. Thus, muscles which become more SO in type might be recruited more readily and so enhance and sustain the spastic state. While this hypothesis may be justified in the early stages, particularly where hypertonus is excessive as in the early head-injured patient, this is rarely apparent in patients with more long standing neurological dysfunction. Over time, the severity of hypertonus often diminishes.

In clinical practice, biomechanical changes in hypertonic muscles occur very rapidly. Muscle stiffness becomes apparent within a short space of time and range of movement is difficult to maintain. Sustained holding in a shortened position can rapidly lead to contracture and this arises as much from active muscle contraction as from poor positioning of limbs (which may be unable to change position because of underlying weakness).[3] Contractures may persist long after the hypertonus resolves and are often responsible for the long standing disability. This is most noticeable in patients following head injury. A year afterwards there may be no evidence of increased tone but the patient is a prisoner within his own body, trapped by residual contractures, making recovering function impossible to utilise. It is therefore impossible to consider the neurological damage which leads to spasticity and secondary changes in muscle properties as separate entities.[26]

Conclusion

Normal movement is the ultimate goal of rehabilitation but all too often, this is not achievable for patients with extensive neurological damage. The analysis of movement described above enables the physiotherapist to select appropriate treatment strategies so that the patient may achieve their optimal level of function. It is not so much a matter of the use of accepted and learned techniques, but more a question of which particular application is appropriate for each individual patient. Compensatory strategies may be necessary for optimal function. The therapeutic skill lies in determining compensation which is necessary and even essential for function, and that which is unnecessary and potentially detrimental to the patient.[10]

The remit of the physiotherapist is also to reduce the effects of the hypertonus and minimise the secondary soft tissue changes. However, the physiotherapist cannot work in isolation. The amount of time which can be spent with any one patient is limited and the beneficial effects of therapy intervention will be short lived if, for the rest of the time, the patient is dominated by the spastic posturing. Treatment plans, devised and implemented in consultation with nursing staff and other healthcare professionals, as well as with relatives and friends, are essential to ensure the continued and ongoing effectiveness of intervention. These must include appropriate positioning and handling and, where indicated, the application and use of splints.

TREATMENT OF THE NEURAL AND BIOMECHANICAL COMPONENTS OF INCREASED TONE

In the light of the above discussion, this section will discuss specific physiotherapy management of patients with increased tone and will include:

- Passive and active movement
- Positioning in lying, sitting and standing
- The use of splinting.

Passive and active movement

Passive joint motion refers to any movement of an articulation that is produced by some external force.[27] It is a potentially dangerous intervention as the patient may be unable to respond appropriately to the forces imposed. This is of particular concern when passive movements are carried out on patients with hypertonus who are dominated by stereotyped posturing which resists movement out of these patterns. Contracture is sometimes complicated by the formation of heterotophic ossification.[28] Vigorous, forceful movements carried out on patients with severe spasticity may cause microtears in muscle which could contribute to calcification.[29]

Specific mobilisation of affected muscle groups is essential to realign and enable more effective movement. Movements should, where possible, be carried out with the patient's active involvement as opposed to passively, or by electrical stimulation. Clearly, this is not always possible but, even if the patient is unconscious, verbal instruction should be given to inform the patient of the desired response and what is expected of him or her. In this way, the maintenance of muscle and joint range becomes a dynamic activity rather than a mindless, routine procedure on the part of both therapist and patient.[30]

Specific attention must be paid to the postural adjustments within the trunk which are essential for providing appropriate background activity for the performance of limb movements. For example, movement of the arm into elevation requires extension of the thoracic spine. This movement will be compromised if spinal mobility is restricted by increased tone. For this reason early mobilisation is advocated where the trunk is accessible, as it is often effective in reducing hypertonus, thereby allowing more selective movement of the limbs. Postural adjustments can also be more accurately monitored.

Muscles which act over more than one joint deserve special consideration. While it may be possible to attain full range of movement at one joint, this is not always so if the muscle is extended throughout its full range. For example, finger extension may be attainable if the wrist is flexed but shortening on the finger flexors is evident when the wrist is extended. This is the basis of the tenodesis grip (Fig. 7.1), whereby the patient relies on tightness of the finger flexors when extending the wrist for hand function. This is a frequent occurrence following spinal cord injury and dependence upon this grip invariably leads to shortening of the finger flexors.

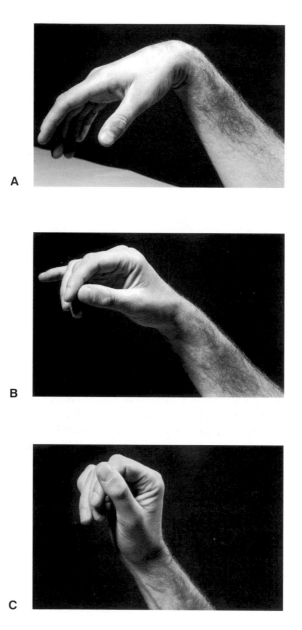

Fig. 7.1   An example of the tenodesis grip in a patient with an incomplete spinal injury at C6 level. Extension of the wrist where there is shortening of the finger flexors allows closure of the hand to form the tenodesis grip (**A**→**C**).

While this is important for effective use of the tenodesis grip, any subsequent recovery in the finger extensors will be compromised by the loss of range into extension.

In summary, emphasis should be placed on active, functional movements with guidance from the physiotherapist to ensure an appropriate response throughout the body as opposed to movement purely at an isolated part. If the patient is unable to participate and, more importantly, is unable to signify pain and discomfort, great care must be taken to prevent overstretching of soft tissue structures and trauma to vulnerable joints.

Positioning

A detailed description of the normal characteristics displayed in various positions can be found elsewhere.[10] Whilst few individuals demonstrate identical characteristics in any given position, certain features are remarkably similar. Table 7.1 provides a summary of these features and, whilst by no means conclusive, it allows comparison to be drawn between normal subjects and those with movement disorders.[20]

Positioning in lying

Generally, in normal subjects, the larger the base of support, the lower the postural tone. However, as noted earlier, in patients with spasticity the tone may actually be increased when lying. Alternative positions may not always be possible, as in the early head-injured patient, and appropriate strategies must be devised to optimise tone management. An example is modified supine lying as illustrated in Fig. 7.2 which may help reduce a dominant extensor pattern. The pillows and wedge positioned under the head and shoulders together with supporting the knees in flexion reduce the tendency for the cervical spine and shoulders to pull back into extension and breaks up the extensor tone in the legs. T-rolls (Fig. 7.3) have also been recommended in that they improve alignment of body segments and thereby symmetry.[32]

Positioning in sitting

Over the past few years, there have been great developments in special seating for people with neurological disability. This is now considered '... a supplement to, or substitute for, mechanisms of

Table 7.1   Characteristics of supported positions and positions requiring anti-gravity activity. Reproduced with permission of the publisher from Edwards S 1998 The incomplete spinal lesion. In: Bromley I (ed) *Tetraplegia and paraplegia: a guide for physiotherapists.* 5th ed. Churchill Livingstone, London.

	Support position		Positions requiring anti-gravity activity		
	Prone	Supine	Supported sitting	Sitting	Standing
Head	To side	Midline	Midline	Midline	Midline
Shoulders	Forwards of CKP	Backwards of CKP	Forwards of CKP	Forwards of CKP	Forwards of CKP
Pelvis	Forwards of CKP (anterior tilt)	Backwards of CKP (posterior tilt)	Forwards of CKP (posterior tilt)	Backwards of CKP (anterior tilt)	Backwards of CKP (posterior tilt)
Upper limbs	Flexion, adduction, medial rotation	Extension, abduction, lateral rotation	Flexion, adduction, medial rotation	Flexion, adduction, medial rotation	Flexion, adduction, medial rotation
Lower limbs	Adduction, medial rotation	Extension, abduction, lateral rotation	Flexion, adduction, medial rotation	Flexion, abduction, lateral rotation	Extension, abduction lateral rotation
Overall influence	Flexion	Extension	Flexion	Flexion	Extension

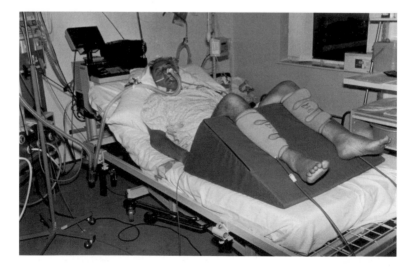

Fig. 7.2   A modified supine position with pillows and wedges to reduce extensor tone. Physiotherapy treatment such as this may be indicated even in the intensive care unit to facilitate nursing care and to prevent soft tissue changes which can develop rapidly.

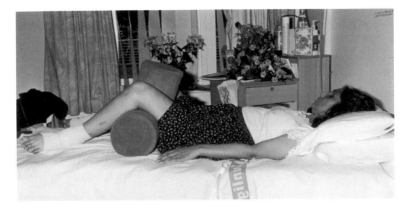

Fig. 7.3   A T-roll placed behind and between the knees can be used to maintain alignment of body segments and improve symmetry.

postural control, with the purpose of reducing the secondary complications associated with the impairment while at the same time facilitating remaining functional ability'.[33]

Many patients with neurological disability demonstrate some degree of postural asymmetry which may be exacerbated by spasticity. It is essential to ensure stability at the hips and pelvis to improve the alignment of body segments and thereby enable more effective movement. Progressive disability may result from poor posturing as the spastic patterning becomes ever more dominant against an inadequate and ineffective base of support. Poor positioning which leaves limbs in shortened positions for prolonged periods must also be avoided to prevent soft tissue changes and contractures.

Wheelchairs and other forms of seating can no longer be viewed as a means of transportation or to enable the patient to be 'sat out'. Many patients spend most of their time in the sitting position and it is essential that seating provision should be individually tailored to the patient's needs to ensure maximum stability and comfort.

Positioning in standing

Standing is advocated as a means of stimulating anti-gravity activity and in maintaining muscle and joint range.[30,34] Different standing aids may be used, the selection of which depends upon the patient's size and weight, medical status and the influence each standing aid has on the postural tone. The more commonly used supports are described elsewhere.[28] These include the tilt table, standing frames of various types (Fig. 7.4), use of back slabs to hold the legs extended and standing the patient between two, or possibly more, physiotherapists or assistants.

Standing is beneficial in that it reduces flexor tone and encourages extensor activity.[28,34] Patients with extensor spasticity may also benefit — ankle plantarflexor tone may be more readily controlled and movements while weight bearing through the feet often serve to reduce tone, not only in the legs but also throughout the rest of the body. Given that shortening of soft tissues occurs so quickly, early standing is recommended for up to half an hour once or twice a day or for as long as the patient can tolerate. The fact that a patient is still unconscious or ventilated need not necessarily preclude this treatment.

One point concerning staff safety. Although having the physiotherapist effect the stand is considered to be a more dynamic intervention than using standing aids, it clearly carries a greater risk for the therapist.

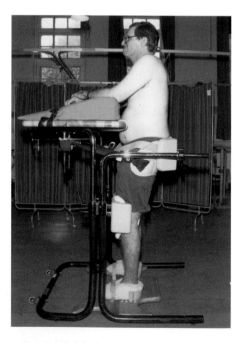

Fig. 7.4   Early standing is advocated to facilitate extension of the lower limbs and reduce flexor tone. Standing frames are valuable aids.

As for walking, opinions differ about the degree of proximal control required before this is undertaken. In the past, some therapists have advocated that the patient must have sufficient proximal control before being allowed to walk. However, it may be argued that the patient is unlikely to develop adequate pelvic and hip control if confined to a wheelchair.

The use of splinting

Many patients with spasticity have affected muscles which are held in a shortened position continuously, either by hypertonia, weakness or poor positioning. Tardieu et al,[35] in a study of children with cerebral palsy, demonstrated that it was necessary for the soleus muscle to remain in a lengthened position for 6 hours to prevent contracture. Physiotherapy may be effective in reducing hypertonia during the course of treatment, but what happens when the patient leaves the treatment area?

The use of splints and orthoses in the management of patients with spasticity is somewhat controversial. Whilst splinting is essential to maintain a prolonged muscle stretch and so prevent contracture, there are some disadvantages. The splinting guidelines produced by the Association of Chartered Physiotherapists Interested in Neurology (ACPIN) provide useful information and recommendations for the appropriate use of splints.[36] Key considerations when electing to splint or not to splint include:

- Is the patient able to accommodate to the splint or does this serve as a resistance against which the patient's spasticity is exacerbated?
- Muscles which are immobilised will atrophy.[24] Do the advantages of maintaining joint range outweigh the effect on muscle?
- Does the use of a splint distally have a positive effect on proximal control or is spasticity 'shunted' to the more proximal muscles?
- What is the purpose of the splint? Is it to maintain range of movement, regain range of movement or to address the problems of muscle imbalance?

Splinting is a useful adjunct to treatment but should not be viewed as a treatment in its own right. A splint will have an effect not only on the part splinted but also on movement in general. For example, a below-knee splint or ankle–foot orthosis (AFO) designed to control the foot in slight dorsiflexion may enable more normal movement at the hip and knee, and thereby a more effective gait. A wrist splint may stabilise the wrist against compensatory flexion at the wrist to allow for improved finger extension.

A combination of 'soft cast' and 'scotch cast' splinting material is increasingly being used in clinical practice.[20] These materials are impregnated with polyurethane resin which sets on exposure to water or air.[37] The scotch cast becomes rigid and the soft cast, semi-rigid. The combination of these two materials allows for specific control across a joint as the clinical presentation dictates. This 'temporary' splinting is recommended to evaluate the effects of a more permanent orthosis. Not only is this beneficial from a therapy perspective but it also allows patients to form their own conclusions as to the effectiveness of the intervention.

Patients with established spasticity may already have loss of muscle and joint range. The shortened muscle may precipitate the spastic response making it even more difficult for the patient to accommodate to the splint. Serial splinting is advocated to regain range of movement,[38] but this is less effective and more time consuming than the use of splints to prevent loss of range.

The use of botulinum toxin to weaken the dominant spastic muscle or muscle group may prove helpful in enabling more effective positioning within the splint. This in turn allows for improved function. For example, in the positive support reaction, botulinum toxin injected into the ankle plantarflexors, in conjunction with a below-knee temporary splint, enables weight bearing through the full surface of the foot as opposed to primarily over the ball of the foot (Fig. 7.5). The weakening of the plantarflexors and the improved alignment of the ankle and foot maintained by the splint, allows for a more fluent and efficient gait pattern.

CONCLUSION

Regenerating axons in the adult CNS are capable of forming synapses with both appropriate and inappropriate target neurones. Facilitation of appropriate patterns of activity will assist in establishing functional connections between regenerating supraspinal axons and spinal neurones.[39] One hypothesis for physiotherapy is that it may encourage this process by facilitating movement to maximise function.

In neurorehabilitation, one of the main aims of physiotherapy is to minimise the effects of spasticity and prevent length-associated changes in muscle to enable more appropriate function. However, while normal movement is the ultimate goal of rehabilitation, all

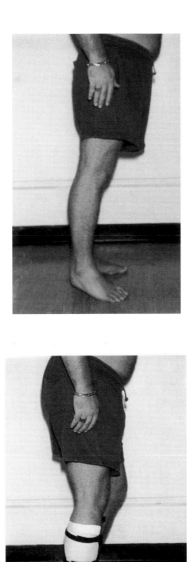

Fig. 7.5   A positive support reaction, involving plantarflexion at the ankle when weight bearing, can be treated with a below-knee splint. Additional focal treatment with botulinum toxin to the plantarflexor muscles may be needed to facilitate this.

too often this is not achievable for patients with extensive neurological damage. There must be a balance between re-education of more normal movement patterns and acceptance, and indeed promotion, of necessary and desirable compensation.[10] The therapeutic skill of the physiotherapist lies in determining the degree of compensation that is necessary and even essential for function, and that which is unnecessary and potentially detrimental to the patient.[20]

REFERENCES

1. Lance JW 1980 Symposium synopsis. In: Feldman RG, Young RR, Koella WP (eds) Spasticity: disordered motor control year book. Year Book Publishers, Chicago, pp 485–494
2. Carr JH, Shepherd RB, Ada L 1995 Spasticity: Research findings and implications for intervention. Physiotherapy 81: 421–429
3. O'Dwyer NJ, Ada L, Neilson PD 1996 Spasticity and muscle contracture following stroke. Brain 119: 1737–1749
4. Dietz V 1992 Human neuronal control of automatic functional movements: interaction between central programs and afferent input. Physiolog Rev 72: 33–69
5. Bobath B 1990 Adult hemiplegia: Evaluation and treatment. 3rd edition. Heinemann Medical Books, Oxford
6. Dattola R, Girlanda P, Vita G, et al 1993 Muscle rearrangement in patients with hemiparesis after stroke: an electrophysiological and morphological study. Eur J Neurol 33: 109–114
7. Herbert R 1988 The passive mechanical properties of muscle and their adaptations to altered patterns of use. Austr J Physiother 34: 141–149
8. Davidoff RA 1992 Skeletal muscle tone and the misunderstood stretch reflex. Neurology 42: 951–963
9. Bernstein N 1967 The co-ordination and regulation of movement. Pergamon, Oxford
10. Edwards S 1996 Analysis of normal movement. In: Edwards S (ed) Neurological physiotherapy: a problem-solving approach. Churchill Livingstone, London, pp 15–40
11. Massion 1992 Movement, posture and equilibrium: interaction and coordination. Prog Neurobiol 38: 35–56
12. Boorman GI, Lee RG, Becker WJ, Windhorst UR 1996 Impaired 'natural reciprocal inhibition' in patients with spasticity due to incomplete spinal cord injury. Electroencephal Clin Neurophysiol 101: 84–92
13. Cordo PJ, Nashner LM 1982 Properties of postural adjustments associated with rapid arm movements. J Neurophysiol 47: 287–302
14. Horak FB, Esselman P, Anderson ME, Lynch MK 1984 The effects of movement velocity, mass displaced, and task certainty on associated postural adjustments made by normal and hemiplegic individuals. J Neurol Neurosurg Psychiatry 47: 1020–1028
15. Rothwell J 1994 Control of human voluntary movement. 2nd edition. Chapman and Hall, London
16. Brooks VB 1986 The neural basis of motor control. Oxford University Press, Oxford
17. Bate P 1997 Motor control theories: insights for therapists. Physiotherapy 83: 397–405

18. Schmidt RA 1991 Motor learning principles for physical therapy. In: Lister M (ed) Contemporary management of motor control problems. Foundation for Physical Therapy, Alexandria, pp 49–63
19. Edwards S 1996 Abnormal tone and movement. In Edwards S (ed) Neurological physiotherapy: a problem-solving approach. Churchill Livingstone, London, pp 63–86
20. Edwards S 1998 The incomplete spinal lesion. In: Bromley I (ed) Tetraplegia and paraplegia: a guide for physiotherapists. 5th edition. Churchill Livingstone, London
21. Shumway-Cook A, Woollacot M 1995 Motor control. Theory and practical applications. Williams and Wilkins, London
22. Henneman E, Somjen G, Carpenter DO 1965 Functional significance of cell size and spinal motoneurones. J Neurophysiol 28: 560–580
23. Goldspink G, Williams P 1990 Muscle fibre and connective tissue changes associated with use and disuse. In: Ada L, Canning C (eds) Key issues in neurological physiotherapy: Physiotherapy foundations for practice. Butterworth Heinemann, Oxford, pp 197–218
24. Given JD, Dewald JPA, Rymer WZ 1995 Joint dependent passive stiffness in paretic and contralateral limbs of spastic patients with hemiparetic stroke. J Neurol Neurosurg Psychiatry 59: 271–279
25. Hufschmidt A, Mauritz K-H 1985 Chronic transformation of muscle in spasticity: a peripheral contribution to increased muscle tone. J Neurol Neurosurg Psychiatry 48: 676–687
26. Nash J, Neilson PD, O'Dwyer NJ 1989 Reducing spasticity to control muscle contracture of children with cerebral palsy. Dev Med Child Neurol 31: 471–480
27. Frank C, Akeson WH, Woo SL-Y Amiel D, Coutts RD 1984 Physiological and therapeutic value of passive joint motion. Clin Orthopaed Rel Res 185: 113–125
28. Edwards S 1996 General principles of treatment. In Edwards S (ed) Neurological physiotherapy: a problem-solving approach. Churchill Livingstone, London, pp 87–113
29. Yarkony G, Sahgal V 1987 Contractures: A major complication of craniocerebral trauma. Clin Orthopaed Related Res 219: 93–96
30. Ada L, Canning C, Paratz J 1990 Care of the unconscious head-injured patient. In: Ada L, Canning C (eds) Key issues in neurological physiotherapy: physiotherapy foundations for practice. Butterworth Heinemann, Oxford, pp 246–286
31. Cosgrove AP, Corry IS, Graham HK 1984 Botulinum toxin in the management of the lower limb in cerebral palsy. Devel Med Child Neurol 36: 386–396
32. Pope P 1992 Management of the physical condition in patients with chronic and severe neurological pathologies. Physiotherapy 78: 896–903
33. Pope P 1996 Postural management and special seating. In Edwards S (ed) Neurological physiotherapy: a problem-solving approach. Churchill Livingstone, London, pp 135–160
34. Brown P 1994 Pathophysiology of spasticity. J Neurol Neurosurg Psychiatry 57: 773–777
35. Tardieu C, Lespargot A, Tarbary C, Bret MD 1988 For how long must the soleus muscle be stretched each day to prevent contracture? Dev Med Child Neurol 30: 3–10
36. Association of Chartered Physiotherapists Interested in Neurology (ACPIN) (in press). Clinical practice guidelines on splinting adults with neurological dysfunction. Chartered Society of Physiotherapy, London
37. Schuren J 1994 Working with soft cast. 3M Minnesota Mining and Manufacturing, Germany
38. Davies PM 1994 Starting again. Springer-Verlag, London
39. Muir GD, Steeves JD 1997 Sensorimotor stimulation to improve locomotor recovery after spinal cord injury. Trends Neurosci 20: 72–77

8. Medical and surgical treatment of spasticity

David J. Werring and Alan J. Thompson

INTRODUCTION

The importance of physiotherapy and patient education in the management of increased tone has been emphasised in previous chapters, and they remain the cornerstone of initial management. However, the increase in our understanding of the normal and disordered functioning of the motor system has provided a number of clinically useful medical and surgical treatments of varying efficacy and invasiveness. To be effective these treatments should be used in conjunction with physiotherapy. This chapter will briefly recap on the pathophysiology and neurochemistry of spasticity underlying the rationale for the various treatments of increased muscle tone. The different methods of influencing activity within the motor system with the aim of reducing tone will then be discussed.

PATHOPHYSIOLOGY OF SPASTICITY

This subject has been discussed in detail in Chapter 3 but a brief summary will be provided here before considering the medical and surgical treatments. Spasticity and many of the associated positive phenomena of the upper motor neurone (UMN) syndrome (Table 1.1) arise principally from disinhibition of spinal reflexes as a result of the UMN lesion. These spinal reflexes include stretch, flexor and extensor reflexes, and are under supraspinal control by inhibitory and excitatory descending pathways. The resulting clinical pattern depends heavily upon the location of the lesion affecting these supraspinal pathways, as well as the speed at which it occurred and the length of time since the lesion. In essence, these clinical phenomena are spinal in origin, arising because of hyperexcitability of the segmental central nervous system (CNS) processing of sensory (afferent) feedback from the periphery. This afferent information includes that from muscle stretch and tension, and from cutaneous (nociceptive and non-nociceptive), joint and visceral (bladder, bowel) stimulation. However, some of the positive phenomena, such as associated reactions and spastic dystonia, may not depend upon sensory feedback and its abnormal processing. These motor overactivities may arise more because of tonic supraspinal drive to the lower motor neurones.

The interneuronal networks governing these spinal reflexes, and the supraspinal pathways that control them, mediate their functions through neurotransmitters, of which there are many (Table 8.1). The main ones appear to be GABA (gamma-aminoburtyric acid), glycine and opioids, which are inhibitory, and excitatory amino acids (EAAs, e.g. glutamate and aspartate), noradrenaline and serotonin, which are excitatory.

THE RATIONALE FOR MEDICAL AND SURGICAL TREATMENT OF SPASTICITY

From the above discussion it can be seen that spasticity, flexor and extensor spasms and so forth depend upon intact neuronal pathways subserving the various spinal reflexes and hyperexcitability of their central processing. There are therefore a variety of theoretical therapeutic strategies which can be targeted at different anatomical sites in the reflex pathways, from the level of spinal segmental interneuronal networks and the synapses, with their descending pathways, to the neuromuscular junction (Fig. 8.1). These strategies range

Table 8.1 Neurotransmitters in the spinal cord. Modified with permission from Advanstar Communications Inc. as reprinted from Neurology®, Nov. 1994, Vol (#44), Number (#11), Supplement (#9), and page (#S12–S20). Neurology® is a registered trademark of the American Academy of Neurology.

Neurotransmitters in descending pathways

Descending pathway	Neurotransmitter
Reticulospinal	Noradrenaline, adrenaline, dopamine, serotonin
Rubrospinal	Excitatory amino acids
Vestibulospinal	Excitatory amino acids
Corticospinal	Glutamate, other excitatory amino acids

Neurotransmitters at spinal segmental level

Activity	Neurotransmitter
Alpha motoneurone collateral	Acetylcholine (nicotinic)
Inhibitory interneuron (Ia)	Glycine
Presynaptic inhibition	GABA
Polysynaptic pathways	Excitatory amino acids, serotonin, substance P, others

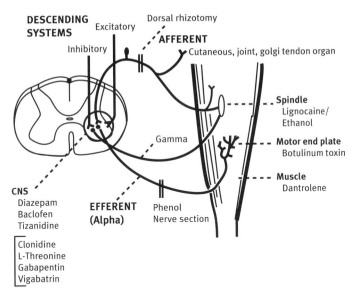

Fig. 8.1   Schematic representation of the spinal cord and reflex arcs indicating points at which therapy may be targeted in the treatment of spasticity.

from pharmacological manipulation of the central neurotransmitters to destructive neurosurgical procedures.

MEDICAL AND SURGICAL TREATMENT OF SPASTICITY

The decision of whether or not to medically treat spasticity has been discussed in detail in Chapter 5. This section will therefore concentrate on the therapies available once this decision has been made. These will be divided into:

- Pharmacological
- Local
- Intrathecal
- Dorsal rhizotomy
- Electrical stimulation.

    Orthopaedic procedures will not be considered.

    In order to optimise their efficacy, treatments for spasticity should not be applied in isolation but must be used in conjunction with physiotherapy, patient education and the removal of exacerbating noxious stimuli where possible.[1]

Pharmacological treatments

As mentioned earlier, the spinal reflexes underlying spasticity and allied phenomena are mediated and controlled by spinal interneurones and by descending pathways, whose influences may be excitatory or inhibitory, and depend on many different neurotransmitters (Table 8.1).[2] Modulation of these neurotransmitters provides the rationale for some of the drug treatments of spasticity, although it should be appreciated that the mechanisms of action even of longstanding treatments such as baclofen are not fully understood. Indeed, three of the most commonly used anti-spasticity treatments, baclofen, diazepam and dantrolene, were discovered serendipitously, before their effects could be described in neuropharmacological or neurophysiological terms.[3] Subsequently, the effects of baclofen, diazepam and, more recently, tizanidine, on various spinal reflex activities have been investigated electrophysiologically and were found to contain differences.[4] While such studies may help to distinguish which patients are most likely to benefit from one drug versus another, the decision currently remains a clinical one. It should be apparent from earlier discussions of pathophysiology (see also Chapter 3) that 'anti-spastic' medications will be beneficial only for those positive phenomena of the UMN syndrome that are mediated by defective control of spinal reflexes (afferent mediated). Some forms of spastic dystonia and associated reactions might well be unaffected, as is often the case clinically.

Of the many oral anti-spastic drugs that have been tried, this section will concentrate primarily on the mainstays of treatment — baclofen, diazepam and dantrolene — as well as a relative newcomer, tizanidine.

Baclofen

For nearly 30 years, baclofen given orally has been known to improve flexor spasms. It is effective even with complete spinal cord transection, so must exert most of its effects at a spinal cord level.[5] Baclofen (beta-4-chlorophenyl-gamma-aminobutyric acid) is structurally related to the inhibitory neurotransmitter GABA, which acts presynaptically to reduce the release of EAAs. Baclofen is an agonist at GABA-B receptors and potentiates this inhibitory effect.[6] In high doses it may also antagonise excitatory neurotransmitters postsynaptically.[7] By virtue of these effects, baclofen may give considerable relief from flexor spasms, whether spontaneous or due to cutaneous stimuli.[8] It may also have a beneficial effect on spastic dystonia in patients with paraplegia or quadriplegia due to spinal cord pathology, notably when due to multiple sclerosis (MS) or traumatic lesions. These actions may have a profound effect on the quality of life of both patient and carers, by relieving pain to allow sleep, and by relaxing leg 'pseudocontractures' to make nursing care and hygiene easier. Although beneficial in spasticity due to cerebral lesions,[9] it appears to be less effective than with spinal causes and is more likely to cause (cognitive) side-effects in this group.

It is usually administered orally and must be started at a low dose which is gradually increased, as tolerated, until the therapeutic response is optimised. A typical starting dose is baclofen 5 mg twice daily, increasing by 5 mg every 3 or 4 days to a maximum dose of about 80 mg daily in divided doses. Once the optimum dose for a given patient is achieved, further increases may diminish the bene-fit obtained. Sudden withdrawal of the drug should be avoided since rebound spasms or, rarely, hallucinations or seizures may result. When used thoughtfully in patients with spinal cord lesions, baclofen has very few serious side-effects. If large doses are given abruptly, especially in those with cerebral lesions, generalised depression of the CNS may result, manifest as sedation, ataxia and cardiorespiratory depression. Hallucinations and confusion may occur in elderly patients, or those with cerebral disease, and an increased seizure frequency has been reported in epileptic patients. In practice, the most common side-effect of baclofen is drowsiness which usually resolves within a few days without the need to reduce the dose. Patients should be advised of the possibility of sedation, particularly with alcohol or other CNS depressants.

Diazepam

Diazepam, like other benzodiazepines, acts by facilitating GABA-mediated inhibition. It does this by increasing the affinity of GABA receptors for the endogenous neurotransmitter, thus enhancing presynaptic inhibition. There may also be an enhancement of endogenous GABA release and a depression of post-synaptic responses to the excitatory transmitter glutamate. Diazepam is use-ful either alone, or in combination with other anti-spasticity agents, in patients with spinal pathology, for example trauma or MS. It is probably less effective than baclofen for intermittent flexor spasms, and may be of more benefit if hypertonia is continuous. It has been shown to be effective for spasticity following complete[10] as well as partial spinal cord lesions, but has not generally been as helpful in spasticity of cerebral origin.

Diazepam should be initiated at a low dose of about 2 mg twice daily, increasing by 2 mg every few days until side-effects become troublesome; particular care should be exercised in the elderly or those with cerebral lesions. The usual maximum dose is about 60 mg daily. The incidence of unwanted side-effects is higher with diazepam than with baclofen. These include somnolence, dizziness and unwanted muscle weakness, and may be exacerbated by CNS depressants including alcohol. In acute overdose coma and respiratory depression can result, so diazepam should be used with caution in those at increased risk of suicide. Paradoxical reactions occasionally occur, including insomnia, anxiety, hostility, hallucinations and increased spasticity. Benzodiazepines also have the capacity to produce physical addiction, and their abrupt withdrawal can precipitate seizures.

Dantrolene

Unlike other anti-spastic drugs, dantrolene acts directly on the contractile apparatus within muscle. It has no specific CNS anti-spastic action, despite side-effects of dizziness and drowsiness. Dantrolene inhibits the release of intramuscular calcium stores from the sarcoplasmic reticulum, which normally follows muscle–membrane depolarisation, and is essential for muscle contraction (excitation–contraction 'uncoupling'). Since it has a peripheral action, it may be used in conjunction with a centrally acting drug. Unfortunately the theoretical benefits of this approach may not be realised since dantrolene can exacerbate some of the side-effects of the centrally acting drug such as drowsiness. Dantrolene has a generalised effect on striated muscle, and so may be particularly helpful in patients whose nursing care is made difficult by prolonged spastic dystonia and who will not be adversely affected by a reduction in voluntary muscle power. It may also have a role if patients are unable to tolerate diazepam or baclofen in adequate dosage because of drowsiness. Dantrolene should be commenced at 25 mg daily, increased by 25 mg every few days (as tolerated) to a maximum of 400 mg daily. As the dose is increased side-effects of nausea, vomiting and muscle weakness will usually be encountered. If no clear clinical benefit is demonstrated within about 6 weeks, therapy should be stopped because of the risk of irreversible liver damage. Liver function tests should be checked before commencing treatment, and subsequently must be closely monitored, particularly in women or the elderly.

Tizanidine

This drug has only just become available in the UK and USA but has been used in the rest of Europe for some time. Its actions are mainly due to an alpha-2 adrenergic receptor agonism, resulting in an inhibitory effect on spinal interneurones of polysynaptic networks.[11] It also has effects on the excitability of the alpha motoneurone, and the descending noradrenergic pathways.[11] It has been claimed that in clinical use tizanidine does not exacerbate or cause muscle weakness in the same way as baclofen or diazepam, but we have yet to confirm this by our own clinical experience. A number of studies have certainly demonstrated a beneficial effect of tizanidine in spasticity due to MS.[12,13] In comparative trials against baclofen, it has demonstrated a similar degree of efficacy.[14,15] A recent randomised, double-blind placebo-controlled study has confirmed this therapeutic benefit in MS patients, and furthermore demonstrated a correlation of effect (as measured by Ashworth Scale change or pendulum test) with plasma concentration.[16] Side-effects of tizanidine include drowsiness and dry mouth, and dose-dependent bradycardia and hypotension.[16] Adverse effects may be minimised by gradual titration of the dose against effects or spreading the dose throughout the day. Tizanidine may also have a specific anti-nociceptive action and some investigators have claimed an improvement in spasticity-associated pain. In summary, tizanidine is a promising new addition to the limited range of helpful therapies for spasticity, with similar efficacy to baclofen and diazepam, but with potentially fewer adverse effects. Its role remains to be established in routine clinical practice.

Clonidine

Clonidine is an antihypertensive which, like tizanidine, is a central alpha-2 adrenergic agonist. It has been shown to be of clinical value in spasticity of both spinal or brainstem origin,[17,18,19] including a reduction in flexor spasms. The mechanism of action is not fully understood, but probably relates to either an inhibitory (presynaptic) effect, possibly on interneurones in the substantia gelatinosa,[17] or by restoring deficient descending pathway noradrenergic inhibition.[20] One study suggested that it may be helpful in patients who fail to respond to baclofen and diazepam.[21]

L-threonine

The amino acid L-threonine is a precursor of glycine, an important post-synaptic inhibitory neurotransmitter in the spinal cord. L-threonine is thought to act as a pro-drug for glycine, which itself is poorly taken up into nervous tissue. L-threonine has achieved modest success in spasticity resulting from familial spastic paraparesis and MS,[22,23] and in spinal spasticity of various causes.[24] However, few patients reported a symptomatic benefit.

Gabapentin

Gabapentin enhances inhibitory GABA-ergic neurotransmission in the CNS. Although it was developed as an anti-epileptic drug, some studies report a benefit in spasticity of spinal origin. One small double-blind, placebo-controlled trial of leg spasticity due to MS[25] found not only a significant improvement in muscle tone, but also in Kurtzke expanded disability status scale (EDSS) scores. Another study of traumatic spinal spasticity found only a modest effect at the standard dose used of 400 mg twice daily.[26] Further studies of gabapentin will be useful in assessing its potential in the treatment of spinal spasticity.

Vigabatrin

Vigabatrin, like gabapentin, is an anti-epileptic that enhances GABA-ergic neurotransmission. It increases GABA concentrations in the CNS by replacing endogenous GABA as a substrate for the catabolic enzyme GABA transaminase. Small studies have shown an improvement in spinal spasticity with similar efficacy to baclofen,[1] and a benefit in spasticity due to a leucodystrophy has also been reported.[27]

Tetrazepam

This benzodiazepine has been studied in a comparative trial with diazepam[28] and was found to exert stronger neurophysiological effects suggesting a more powerful effect on presynaptic inhibition. It was also found to be better tolerated. Further clinical studies are required to determine whether or not tetrazepam will have a useful therapeutic role in spasticity.

Orphenadrine

Orphenadrine blocks muscarinic acetylcholine receptors, and has been used to treat parkinsonism. A double-blind, placebo-controlled trial in patients with spinal cord injury has reported a beneficial effect[29] on both neurophysiological and clinical findings.

Other drug treatments

There have been well-publicised anecdotal reports of benefit from cannabinoids in alleviating spasticity in MS, and some limited data from clinical trials.[30] The cognitive and affective side-effects of cannabinoids are unfortunately likely to be particularly pronounced in patients with MS, in whom cognitive deficits are common. There is a great deal of interest in the development of new drugs designed to modulate the effects of neurotransmitters at a spinal level, particularly glutamate antagonists.[2] The neurotransmitters for the relevant interneuronal circuits in the spinal cord need to be identified to facilitate a comprehensive and rational approach to pharmacological interventions.

Local treatments

Phenol

Phenol is a neurolytic agent that impairs nerve conduction when injected in close proximity to peripheral nerves. The effect on spasticity is often immediate, generally longer lasting than that of botulinum toxin (BTX), and may be permanent. Furthermore the injections are non-selective, causing damage to both motor and sensory nerves in the vicinity. For these reasons, electromyography (EMG) guidance is desirable. A number of peripheral nerves in the upper and lower limb are amenable to phenol injections and treatment applied to each nerve may reduce specific patterns of spasticity and functional loss. For example, the injection of the sciatic nerve may reduce hamstring spasticity, thus helping with seating and positioning, aiding gait and transfers, and preventing pressure sores. Some of the undesirable effects of phenol include painful dysaesthesiae and a highly variable and unpredictable duration of effect. For a more detailed review the interested reader is directed to Skeil and Barnes.[31]

Botulinum toxin

For many years BTX has been the treatment of choice for a number of focal dystonias,[32] but has only recently come to prominence as a treatment for spasticity. It functionally denervates a muscle through neuromuscular junction blockade and is a uniquely targeted and specific method of reducing muscle activity. Botulinum toxin has been reported to increase range of movement in spasticity at the elbow, wrist and fingers,[33] and has also been shown to reduce adductor spasms in patients with MS.[34] In our unit we have shown a benefit from botulinum injection on distal limb spasticity, as exemplified by the improvement in hand function in a patient with an incomplete traumatic cervical spinal cord injury;[35] we are currently engaged in a randomised, double-blind, placebo-controlled trial of BTX in the treatment of upper and lower limb spasticity. Botulinum toxin is discussed in more detail in Chapter 9.

Lignocaine/ethanol

Intramuscular administration of lignocaine or ethanol have been used in an attempt to induce a blockade of Ia muscle afferent fibres arising from the muscle spindle. In one study, this 'muscle afferent block' was found to have a beneficial effect comparable to that obtained with BTX in a variety of lower and upper limb spasticity patterns.[36] Duration of effect was initially very short (less than 24 hours), but with repeated injections every 3–4 days this was prolonged to several weeks. This treatment may be a useful and less costly alternative to other focal treatments.

Intrathecal treatments

Phenol

Although phenol is currently used mainly to block peripheral nerves, the first reported use in spasticity was via the intrathecal route.[37,38] Intrathecal phenol has become less popular, partly due to its well-recognised adverse effects and partly due to the recent advent of intrathecal baclofen. Intrathecal phenol often damages the sacral nerves which may result in faecal and urinary incontinence, and may occasionally also damage sympathetic nerves resulting in abnormal vasomotor responses and pressure sores. However, it is a relatively simple practical procedure which may be very effective in patients who are severely disabled with pre-existing loss of bladder and bowel function, and who are not able to tolerate the more technically complex treatment of intrathecal baclofen.

Baclofen

A relatively recent advance in spasticity management has been the administration of baclofen by the intrathecal route using an implanted pump.[39] This has a potent theoretical advantage over the oral route: the catheter may be placed to maximise drug delivery to the appropriate region of the neuraxis (lumbar spinal cord), with a consequent increase in efficacy and reduction in systemic side-effects from a given dose. Very small doses may be used since many GABA receptors are located in the superficial laminae of the spinal cord and are therefore readily accessible to cerebrospinal fluid (CSF). These benefits have been translated into clinical practice in patients with severe spinal spasticity refractory to oral treatments.[40, 41] A randomised, double-blind, placebo-controlled trial with 93 cases of intractable spasticity due to spinal cord injury or MS showed a reduction in muscle rigidity and spasms with minimal adverse effects. [42] Intrathecal baclofen has also been shown to be of some value in patients with severe spasticity from traumatic or hypoxic brain injury,[43] suggesting that its use may not be confined to the treatment of spinal pathology.

Baclofen is administered intrathecally by means of an implantable subcutaneous pump combining a reservoir and delivery mechanism.[44] The pump is connected via a catheter tunnelled under the skin to the L3–L4 intrathecal space. Modern devices are externally programmable, allowing titration of dose whilst the pump remains *in situ*.

The selection of patients for intrathecal baclofen requires careful consideration. Some suggested criteria are presented in Table 8.2.[44]

Table 8.2   Suggested criteria for selecting patients for intrathecal baclofen. Modified with permission of the publisher, Mark Allen Publishing Ltd, from McLean BN 1993 intrathecal baclofen in severe spasticity. British J Hosp Med 49: 262–267.

- Spasticity resulting in severe functional disability or pain
- Non-progressive or slowly progressive causes of spasticity, including trauma, multiple sclerosis or cerebral palsy
- Oral medication is ineffective or associated with intolerable side-effects
- Patients and carer(s) are capable of practically dealing with pump, including attendance for regular review of efficacy, adverse effects and maintenance
- Patients and carer(s) are capable of understanding the risks involved

Dorsal rhizotomy

Surgical anterior and posterior rhizotomy have been used for many years for intractable spasticity, but more selective procedures are now possible. Microsurgical lesions of the dorsal root entry zone (DREZ) of the lateral root destroy small nociceptive afferents whilst sparing large fibres. This should preferentially remove the input from nociceptors and muscle spindles, thus reducing flexor and stretch reflexes without complete limb deafferentation.[45] The procedure may relieve both pain and spasticity, but is clearly irreversible and carries a surgical risk. The less invasive technique of percutaneous radiofrequency rhizotomy has been reported to be effective with minimal risk to sphincter or sexual function.[46] The more selective approaches outlined here have now largely replaced the older, more destructive procedures of cordotomies, neurectomies and rhizotomies, and retain a useful but limited role in clinical practice.

Electrical stimulation

A rectal electrostimulation probe has been successfully used to relieve painful spasms and hypertonia in paraplegia for between 3 and 24 hours,[47] although the benefit was not as marked as that resulting from intrathecal baclofen. The mode of action is not known but probably relates to the stimulation of perineal afferent fibres. A significant side-effect is autonomic dysreflexia.

Chronic dorsal column stimulation using an implanted electrode has been reported to be of value in spasticity,[48] but is not clearly established to be of benefit.

Practical approach to the treatment of spasticity

The selection of patients for drug treatment remains clinical and patients with disabling increased tone or spasms, with or without pain, merit consideration. The first clinical point to establish prior to treatment is whether the spasticity is generalised or focal. If the problem is generalised (i.e. affecting more than one limb) then it is reasonable to consider systemic drug treatment. If there is a clearly identifiable focal component, such as involuntary wrist or finger flexion, then it may be appropriate to first consider a focal treatment, for example BTX injections. As emphasised previously, exacerbating stimuli should be carefully sought and eliminated if possible. Physiotherapy must be involved as soon as possible to maximise functional recovery and minimise the development of irreversible contractures.

The choice of a first-line oral agent lies between baclofen and diazepam. If spasms are painful and severe then baclofen should be initiated at first, with careful titration of the dosage until benefit is obtained or side-effects (e.g. drowsiness) are experienced. The benefit is usually judged from the subjective impression of the patient, carers and therapists as objective outcome measures are often not used routinely. As such, it is often difficult to make a firm conclusion regarding efficacy and for this reason a trial of drug withdrawal may clarify the situation. The anti-spastic efficacy of baclofen is similar to that of diazepam, but it has the important advantage of causing less sedation or reduction in voluntary muscle power. Unlike dantrolene it is also free of side-effects on other organ systems. If clear benefit has not been shown with baclofen, diazepam may be substituted or added. In our experience it has limited value in a small dose as an adjunct to baclofen, although drowsiness or muscle weakness may result.

Patients often express concern regarding the addictive potential of benzodiazepines, which in practice may limit their use. The newer agent tizanidine may be an appropriate choice if muscle weakness is a problem with baclofen or diazepam, and is preferable to dantrolene because of its better safety profile.

If none of these agents — baclofen, diazepam or tizanidine — are effective then dantrolene may be considered, but only in patients with normal liver function. The risk of irreversible liver damage necessitates the regular monitoring of plasma liver enzymes. There is certainly a theoretical argument for combining a central agent (baclofen or diazepam) with the peripherally acting dantrolene, but the combination in practice is often poorly tolerated as dantrolene has some CNS side-effects. All of the agents mentioned above have potentially serious side-effects and their continuation should always be based on clearly demonstrated clinical benefit.

If these agents are not helpful then the 'second-line' treatments clonidine, L-threonine, vigabatrin and gabapentin could be considered. Clinical experience with these drugs is very limited and the effects of long-term administration are not known. If treatment is not effective using a single oral agent, then it is reasonable to try a combination of drugs with different modes of action in the hope of achieving a synergistic effect. Before embarking on this strategy, a single agent should have been tried at the maximum tolerable dose since the principle of keeping treatment as simple as possible holds for spasticity in the same way as in medical therapeutics generally. In our experience, if spasticity is so severe that a single agent has no effect even at a high dose then it is unlikely to respond to two or more drugs. At this stage more invasive treatments may be considered.

If the refractory spasticity is focal, then it is better to employ BTX or phenol in preference to intrathecal treatments. There are varying views regarding the optimal invasive treatment of a spastic paraparesis. There are arguments in favour of either botulinum injections to the adductor muscles or intrathecal baclofen in this situation and both treatments have been shown to be effective. The temporary action of BTX, requiring repeated injections every 3 months or so, may be seen as a drawback. However, an intrathecal baclofen pump also requires regular maintenance and refilling or dosage adjustment, also necessitating a return to the treating hospital every 3 months or so.

The first-line invasive treatment for generalised spasticity should probably be intrathecal baclofen, whose value has been clearly shown in a large number of clinical trials. A number of criteria should be fulfilled before commencing a trial of intrathecal baclofen, some of which have already been discussed (Table 8.2). The patient should be able to give informed consent and should understand the basic principles of the treatment. Spasticity should normally be of spinal origin, long-standing (more than 1 year), non-progressive and not manageable with oral drugs (including baclofen). There should be a definite response to a test dose of intrathecal baclofen demonstrated before a permanent pump is inserted. If intrathecal baclofen is not effective then other invasive or more experimental treatments may be considered. These include BTX, nerve blocks and electrical stimulation. We would recommend BTX first, since it is generally safe, well tolerated and reversible. As clinical experience with BTX increases, its use in routine clinical management of spasticity is also likely to increase, particularly in the treatment of focal abnormalities.

CONCLUSION

This chapter has discussed some of the available medical and surgical options for the treatment of spasticity. We have attempted to provide a rationale for the use of these treatments by placing them in a pathophysiological context. We have emphasised the need for integration with physiotherapy, which remains a most important part of any treatment regimen for spasticity. The need to seek potential exacerbating factors before commencing any treatment has also been stressed. A practical approach to using the available treatments has been suggested, beginning with the longest-established oral agents and moving onwards to more experimental or invasive therapies if these are ineffective.

REFERENCES

1. Losseff N, Thompson AJ 1995 The medical management of increased tone. Physiotherapy 81: 480–484
2. Young RR 1994 Spasticity: a review. Neurology 44 (suppl 9): S12-S20
3. Young RR 1980 Treatment of spastic paraparesis. N Engl J Med 320: 1553–1555
4. Delwaide PJ, Pennisi G 1994 Tizanidine and electrophysiologic analysis of spinal control mechanisms in humans with spasticity. Neurology 44 (suppl 9): S21-S28
5. Pederson E, Arlien-Soborg P, Mai J 1974 The mode of action of the GABA derivative baclofen in human spasticity. Acta Neurol Scand 50: 665–680
6. Hwang AS, Wilcox GL 1989 Baclofen, gamma-aminobutyric acid B receptors and substance P in the mouse spinal cord. J Pharmacol Exp Ther 248: 1026–1033
7. Blaxter TJ, Carlen PL 1985 Pre- and postsynaptic effects of baclofen in the rat hippocampal slice. Brain Res 341: 195–199
8. Duncan GW, Shahani BT, Young RR 1976 An evaluation of baclofen for certain symptoms in patients with spinal cord lesions: a double-blind cross-over study. Neurology 26: 441–446
9. van Hemert JCJ 1980 Pathophysiology of spasticity and clinical experience with baclofen. In: Feldman RG, Young RR, Koella WP (eds) Spasticity: disordered motor control. Year Book Medical Publishers, Chicago, pp 41–49
10. Corbett M, Frankel HL, Michaelis L 1972 A double-blind, cross-over trial of Valium in the treatment of spasticity. Paraplegia 10: 19–22
11. Wagstaff AJ, Bryson HM 1997 Tizanidine. A review of its pharmacology, clinical efficacy and tolerability in the management of spasticity associated with cerebral and spinal disorders. Drugs 53: 435–452
12. Emre M, Leslie M, Muir C, et al 1994 Correlations between dose, plasma concentrations and antispastic action of tizanidine. J Neurol Neurosurg Psychiatry 57: 1355–1359
13. The United Kingdom Tizanidine Trial Group 1994 A double-blind, placebo-controlled trial of tizanidine in the treatment of spasticity caused by multiple sclerosis. Neurology 44 (suppl 9): S70–S78
14. Hassan N, McLellan DL 1980 Double-blind comparison of single doses of DS 103–282, baclofen and placebo for suppression of spasticity. J Neurol Neurosurg Psychiatry 43: 1132–1136
15. Hoogstraten MC, van der Ploeg RJO, van der Burg W, et al 1988 Tizanidine versus baclofen in the treatment of spasticity in multiple sclerosis patients. Acta Neurol Scand 77: 224–230
16. Nance PW, Sheremata WA, Lynch SG, et al 1997 Relationship of the antispasticity effect of tizanidine to plasma concentration in patients with multiple sclerosis. Arch Neurol 54: 731–736
17. Donovan WH, Carter RE, Rossi CD, Wilerson MA 1988 Clonidine effect on spasticity: a clinical trial. Arch Phys Med Rehabil 69: 193–195
18. Maynard FM 1986 Early clinical experience with clonidine in spinal spasticity. Paraplegia 24: 175–182

19. Sanford PR, Spengler SE, Sawasky KB 1992 Clonidine in the treatment of brainstem spasticity. Am J Phys Med Rehabil 71: 301–303
20. Nance PW, Shears AH, Nance DM 1989 Reflex change induced by clonidine in spinal cord injured patients. Paraplegia 27: 296–301
21. Khan O, Olek MJ 1995 Clonidine in the treatment of spasticity in patients with multiple sclerosis. J Neurol 242: 712–715
22. Growden JH, Nader TM, Schoenfield J, Wurtman RJ 1991 L-threonine in the treatment of spasticity. Clin Neuropharm 14: 403–412
23. Hauser SL, Doolittle TH, Lopez-Bresnahan M, et al 1992 An antispastic effect of threonine in multiple sclerosis. Arch Neurol 49: 923–926
24. Lee A, Patterson V 1993 A double-blind study of L-threonine in patients with spinal spasticity. Acta Neurol Scand 88: 334–338
25. Mueller ME, Gruenthal M, Olson WL, Olson WH 1997 Gabapentin for relief of upper motoneuron symptoms in multiple sclerosis. Arch Phys Med Rehabil 78: 521–524
26. Priebe MM, Sherwood AM, Graves DE, Mueller M, Olson WH 1997 Effectiveness of gabapentin in controlling spasticity: a quantitative study. Spinal Cord 35: 171–175
27. Jaeken J, DeCock P, Casaer P 1991 Vigabatrin as a spasmolytic drug. Lancet 338: 8782–8783
28. Delwaide PJ, Pennisi G 1997 A comparative electrophysiologic study of diazepam and tetrazepam in patients with spasticity. J Neurol Rehabil 11: 91–96
29. Casale R, Glynn CJ, Buonocore M 1995 Reduction of spastic hypertonia in patients with spinal cord injury. A double-blind comparison of IV orphenadrine citrate and placebo. Arch Phys Med Rehabil 76: 660–665
30. Petro DJ, Ellenberger C 1981 Treatment of human spasticity with delta-9-tetrahydrocannabinol. J Clin Pharmacol 21: 413–416
31. Skeil DA, Barnes MP 1994 The local treatment of spasticity. Clin Rehabil 8: 240–246
32. Jankovic J, Brin MF 1991 The therapeutic uses of botulinum toxin. N Engl J Med 324: 1186–1194
33. Das TK, Park DM 1989 Effect of treatment with botulinum toxin on spasticity. Postgrad Med J 65: 208–210
34. Snow BJ, Tsui JKC, Batt MH 1990 Treatment of spasticity with botulinum toxin: a double-blind study. Ann Neurol 28: 512–515
35. Richardson D, Edwards S, Sheean GL, Greenwood RJ, Thompson AJ 1997 The effect of botulinum toxin on hand function after incomplete spinal cord injury at the level of C5-C6: a case report. Clin Rehabil 11: 288–292
36. Kaji R, Mezaki T, Kubori T, Murase N, Kimura J 1996 Treatment of spasticity with botulinum toxin and muscle afferent block. Clin Neurol 36: 1334–1335
37. Kelly RE, Gautier-Smith PC 1959 Intrathecal phenol in the treatment of reflex spasms and spasticity. Lancet ii: 1102–1105
38. Nathan PW 1959 Intrathecal phenol to relieve spasticity in paraplegia. Lancet ii: 1099–1102
39. Penn RD and Kroin JS 1984 Intrathecal baclofen alleviates spinal cord spasticity. Lancet i: 1078
40. Penn RD, Savoy SM, Corcos D, et al 1989 Intrathecal baclofen for severe spinal spasticity. N Engl J Med 320: 1517–1521
41. Ochs G, Struppler A, Meyerson BA, et al 1989 Intrathecal baclofen for long-term treatment of spasticity: A multi-centre study. J Neurol Neurosurg Psychiatry 52: 933–939
42. Coffey RJ, Cahill D, Steers W, et al 1993 Intrathecal baclofen for intractable spasticity of spinal origin: results of a long-term multicenter study. J Neurosurg 78: 226–232

43. Becker R, Alberti O, Bauer BL 1997 Continuous intrathecal baclofen in severe spasticity after traumatic or hypoxic brain injury. J Neurol 244: 160–166
44. McLean BN 1993 Intrathecal baclofen in severe spasticity. British J Hosp Med 49: 262–267
45. Sindou M 1989 Microsurgical DREZ-tomy for the treatment of pain and spasticity In: Young RR, Delwaide PJ (eds). Principles and practice of restorative neurology. Oxford, Butterworth/Heinemann, 144–151
46. Kasdon DL, Lathi ES 1984 A prospective study of radiofrequency rhizotomy in the treatment of post-traumatic spasticity. Neurosurgery 15: 526–529
47. Halstead LS, Seager SWJ, Houston JM, et al 1993 Relief of spasticity in SCI men and women using rectal probe electrostimulation. Paraplegia 31: 715–721
48. McBride GG 1993 Dorsal column stimulation to control severe spasticity in spinal cord injury patients. J Am Paraplegia Soc 16: 134

9. The treatment of spasticity with botulinum toxin

Geoffrey L. Sheean

INTRODUCTION

It is clear from the previous chapter that there is often a need for focal treatment of motor overactivity in the upper motor neurone (UMN) syndrome. This chapter will discuss the rationale for the use of botulinum toxin (BTX) in this situation followed by an overview of the relevant literature pertaining to this use. The management procedure practiced at The National Hospital for Neurology and Neurosurgery will be outlined, with attention to the practical details. Case histories will be used to illustrate some of the points.

NEED FOR FOCAL TREATMENT

As the preceding chapters indicate, medical anti-spastic therapy, by its systemic nature, is non-focal or global in its effects. As a result, the dose required to reduce motor activity in the desired area may produce relative hypotonia or weakness elsewhere that is functionally detrimental. For example, treating a strong plantarflexion response when standing with oral baclofen may reduce muscle tone throughout the whole leg, making it more difficult to stand. Additional drawbacks of medical therapy include difficulty in titrating the clinical effect and systemic side-effects.

Physiotherapists have a variety of methods to reduce motor over-activity in focal areas, as outlined in Chapter 7. However, sometimes these methods fail or produce results too slowly and additional treatment is needed. Until recently, the only focal treatments were phenol injections and surgery; both have serious drawbacks (Chapter 8). When BTX was introduced for focal dystonia, it was not long before its potential to reduce focal 'spasticity' was recognised.

the muscle becomes functionally 'denervated'. The exact site of action within the presynaptic nerve terminal varies with the serotype of BTX (for review see Dolly[2]). The only commercially available serotype, BTX Type A, binds irreversibly to an ACh vesicle binding protein called SNAP-25. Recovery from the blockade occurs via the sprouting of new axons from adjacent nerves, as well as from the pre-terminal portions of the affected nerves, and takes about 3 months. In this time, the muscle is weak and may atrophy. Electromyography (EMG) may reveal denervation potentials (fibrillations and positive sharp waves) and the motor units appear more 'myopathic', rather than neurogenic. This is because the toxin blocks neuromuscular junctions of individual muscle fibres, functionally denervating each one, rather than a whole motor unit.

The clinical benefit is thought to arise from this neuromuscular junction blockade and associated weakness. It has been speculated that other mechanisms may also contribute, such as a CNS action and an effect on gamma fusimotor fibres at the level of the muscle spindle. There is some evidence to support the latter[3] but no convincing evidence that BTX has a direct effect on the CNS. Nonetheless, many patients with dystonia seem to derive enormous benefit from very little weakness and others have a clinical response well outlasting the weakness. The latter could be understandable in the UMN syndrome if, during the period of weakness, substantial gains were made that were contributed to and sustained by physical therapy.

EXPERIENCE WITH BTX IN SPASTICITY

Literature review

There have been a large number of uncontrolled and a smaller number of placebo-controlled trials[4-7] of the use of BTX in adult 'spasticity', the results of which have been summarised by O'Brien.[8] Considering just the placebo-controlled trials, these have generally dealt with hypertonia, assumed to be spasticity, arising from stroke, multiple sclerosis (MS) or head injury. Muscles injected included thigh adductors,[4] ankle plantarflexors and invertors,[6] elbow and wrist flexors,[7] or various muscles.[5] EMG was not always performed to ensure that the hypertonia and reduced range of movement was due to muscular overactivity. Overall, there is a clear result that BTX can reduce tone and increase range of movement for a period of time — usually 2–6 months[8] — similar to dystonia. This outcome should not be at all surprising as it is merely stating that given a sufficient dose of BTX, overactive muscles can be weakened. However, these trials have provided a guide to the effective doses.

What has not yet been fully substantiated is that this reduction in tone and increased range of movement produces some positive benefit for the patient, particularly in terms of active function. Many studies have reported improvement in gait or hand function for some patients as well as a reduction in pain, subjective improvements in ease of caring for the patient in performing physiotherapy, among others. This is in contrast with studies of cerebral palsy in children where a clear functional benefit (improved gait) can be obtained.[9] As discussed in earlier chapters, the likelihood of showing a functional gain from BTX will depend upon whether or not the assumption that the motor overactivity being treated was contributing significantly to the functional loss is correct. The same question applies equally well to any anti-spastic treatment, focal or otherwise. Our own clinical experience shows us that functional goals are achievable in *selected* patients. Patient selection remains the key to success and rests heavily on the aforementioned assumption being correct. The many complex factors involved in the selection process will probably make design of controlled trials to examine the functional benefits of BTX extremely difficult, if not impossible. Such information will probably have to come from subjective reports of the collective experience of expert centres.

CLINICAL APPROACH TO TREATMENT WITH BTX

The following sections are based upon our own experience of treating patients with BTX and cannot be supported by data from rigorous trials. Discussion with other centres suggests that our clinical approaches and experiences are similar. The management of spasticity and other features of the UMN syndrome with BTX can be divided into several steps:

1. Identification of clinical problem
2. Evaluation of clinical problem
3. Setting treatment goals and injection schedule
4. Select outcome measurement
5. Injection procedure
6. Post-injection physiotherapy and follow-up.

Identification of clinical problem

Indications for BTX in the UMN syndrome

Treatment with BTX should be considered when there is a clinical problem arising directly or indirectly from focal excessive or inappropriate muscular contraction. Referring back to the flow-chart of clinical problems in the UMN syndrome (Fig. 2.2), such clinical problems can be grouped broadly into (Table 9.2):

1. Pain
2. Restriction of movement
3. Excessive/inappropriate movement.

These have more advanced consequences. All three may interfere with function (both active and passive) and impair physical therapy while the first may also lead to skin damage, e.g. in the palm and intertrigonous areas. Restriction of movement may lead to a fixed posture and secondary soft tissue changes which may lead to irreversible muscle contractures. Common clinical problems are listed in Table 9.3.

The mainstay of treatment is physical therapy, with or without oral medications, and should be continued even if BTX is added. BTX is usually second line, to be considered if the problem is either not responding to adequate physiotherapy or was responding too slowly. We do not inject patients without them having first received an adequate period of intensive physiotherapy. As with all spasticity treatments, any aggravating factors should be eliminated first (Table 5.2). One patient was rejected because of a painful ulcer on the 'spastic' leg which, when treated, reduced the spasticity and obviated the need for BTX injection.

Table 9.2 Common basic forms of motor overactivity treated with botulinum toxin

Restriction of movement	Excessive/inappropriate movement
Flexed fingers or wrist	Spasms – flexor, extensor
Flexed elbow	Positive support reaction
Adducted hips	Ankle clonus
Flexed knee	Extensor toe
	Associated reaction (elbow flexion)

Table 9.3   Common adverse consequences of motor overactivity treated with botulinum toxin

- Pain
- Development of soft tissue changes
- Skin damage
- Posture threatening tracheostomy (elbow flexion)
- Interference with gait
- Interference with hand function
- Impairment of physiotherapy procedures (splinting, casting, orthoses)
- Difficulty nursing patient (abnormal posture)

Evaluation of clinical problem

A multidisciplinary approach

We strongly advocate a multidisciplinary approach when assessing the need for BTX injections, utilizing the specialist services of a neurologist/neurorehabilitationist, physiotherapist and clinical neurophysiologist. Expert physiotherapy assessment is invaluable for the therapist's knowledge of functional anatomy and the dynamics of normal movement. As with oral anti-spastic therapy, the therapist can predict the consequences of weakening muscles, thus helping to avoid a deterioration of function from excessive or inappropriate weakness. Physiotherapists also play an essential role in follow-up therapy (stretching, splinting, and casting – see Chapter 7) and in the application of outcome measures to monitor the clinical response. The neurologist/neurorehabilitationist guides therapy and integrates BTX injections with other medical treatments. Finally, the clinical neurophysiologist contributes to both assessment and injection through EMG. All of this is quite time-consuming (about 30 minutes for a new case) and labour intensive but quite necessary as we believe that the key to success with BTX treatment is in careful patient assessment and selection.

EMG assessment

EMG assessment before BTX injection can be helpful in several ways. It can help establish the relative contributions of neural and biomechanical components to the hypertonia. Hypertonia, predominantly due to soft tissue changes, is unsuitable for BTX injections; treatment should focus more on physical therapy. Secondly, it can identify the overactive muscles as not all agonists may behave the same. For example, in one patient with marked hypertonia of the elbow flexors, biceps exhibited little EMG activity during passive stretch whereas brachialis and brachioradialis were contracting very actively. Such information can help determine the target muscles and doses for injection based upon the degree of active muscle contraction seen. Thirdly, EMG can give some idea of the strength of voluntary activity, particularly of antagonists. For example, a patient with marked hypertonia in the finger flexors may show no active finger extension, but EMG may show active recruitment of motor units in the finger extensors, indicating some preservation of voluntary strength. The advantages of EMG in performing the injection will be discussed later.

We look for the presence of EMG activity at rest and in response to a passive stretch of the muscles. This stretch is performed at different velocities to identify spasticity, a velocity-dependent, kinetic stretch response. Sustained stretches are also given to look for a static stretch response and the stretch is maintained to observe for any fatigue of the response. Such fatigue would encourage the use of splinting to maintain length and reduce the stretch response; the absence of fatigue might suggest that splinting would be unsuccessful. Stretch responses may also fatigue with repeated stretches, also encouraging for splinting. Determining the relative proportions of soft tissue change and active muscle contraction in the production of hypertonia is particularly difficult. An experienced electromyographer can do this by comparing the resistance felt to passive movement and the EMG interference pattern (i.e. amount of EMG activity). The patterns of EMG activity that may be encountered are illustrated in Fig. 9.2. In many cases, a dynamic recording during standing or walking may be necessary as there may be no abnormal activity at rest or in response to stretch.

Setting treatment goals and injection schedule

The ultimate goals of therapy with BTX are no different to those of spasticity treatment in general, nor to the specific goals of other focal treatments such as physical therapy and phenol nerve blocks. The process of setting treatment goals and choosing outcome measures has been discussed in Chapter 6. The very basic, level one treatment goal of BTX is to produce an adequate, but not excessive, weakening of the muscle and reduction in tone.

Common examples of goals of BTX treatment are given in Table 9.4. The patients should be reminded that the injections actually

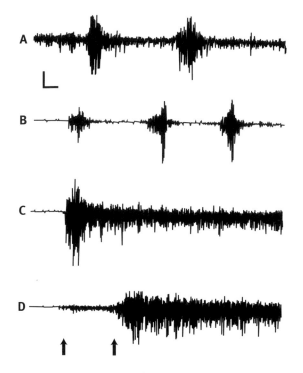

Fig. 9.2   Examples of EMG patterns that may be seen in the UMN syndrome. **A.** Tonic activity at rest with bursts of activity in response to rapid stretches; **B.** Spasticity — bursts of EMG activity during rapid stretches representing dynamic tonic stretch reflexes; **C.** A static stretch response — after an initial burst, the EMG activity is maintained as long as the stretch is sustained; **D.** EMG activity in plantarflexors during attempted movement only (a positive support reaction) — no EMG activity when sitting, a small amount when standing without weight bearing (first arrow) and a marked increase when weight bearing (second arrow). Calibration 500 mV, 500 ms.

weaken muscles and are not going to make them stronger. Achieving a functional goal depends upon many factors, such as:

- The presence of a clear functional goal
- Functional disability being largely due to focal motor over-activity
- Preservation of some agonist–antagonist function[8]
- Minimal disability due to neurological deficits (e.g. weakness, apraxia, sensory loss)
- Continuing active physiotherapy after injection
- Patient factors — motivation, cognition, general health.

Table 9.4 Common botulinum toxin treatment goals

Symptomatic	Functional (neurorehabilitative)
Reduce pain and spasms	Hand function – reach, grasp and carry
Improve passive range of movement	Standing and gait
Improve hygiene – palm, intertriginous area	
Assist nursing/self-care – dressing, feeding, bathing, self-catheterisation	

Probably the two most important factors are, the correct assumption that functional disability is being contributed to substantially by motor overactivity, and the preservation of some agonist and antagonist function.

Contraindications to BTX treatment are largely relative, the presence of a substantial soft tissue component to hypertonia and a lack of physiotherapy follow-up being two of the more important. Fixed contracture has been cited as a contraindication, but such patients may still be troubled by superimposed muscle spasms which respond to BTX. Some muscles are difficult and potentially risky to inject, such as hip flexors, and injection should be carefully considered.

The expected treatment schedule depends largely upon the basic goal of therapy. A long-term schedule of repeated injections indefinitely assumes that the course of the condition is static and will not be changed either by the injection or accompanying physical therapies. The benefits of the injection are not sustained and treatment with BTX in this way is similar to that of dystonia, where BTX is the main therapy. In contrast, the short-term schedule of only a few injections assumes that the course of the condition is towards progressive improvement. This occurs either naturally or as a result of the treatment given and is a more neurorehabilitative approach than the first. Thus, neurorehabilitative physical therapy is the main treatment and BTX is an adjunct. One situation demanding a short-term treatment schedule might be that of marked (neural) hypertonia appearing soon after a head injury. This hypertonia may last only a few weeks, but in that time secondary soft tissue changes and contracture can appear. When natural recovery occurs and the motor overactivity has subsided, the patients finds themselves severely disabled by the often refractory soft tissue changes that might have been avoided by early use of BTX.

When used as a short-term adjunct to therapy, it is assumed that any benefits obtained from BTX will be sustained. While it is possible that BTX can directly affect the basic pathophysiological process to produce a sustained reduction in motor overactivity, it is more likely that a sustained benefit arises either from natural recovery or from the physical therapy itself. One of the basic goals of physical therapy is to maximise and maintain muscle length and range of movement (ROM). This both reduces and prevents soft tissue changes, as well as reducing excitability of the tonic stretch reflex, that is, reducing spasticity. By producing short-term weakness of the overactive muscles, BTX produces a short-term gain (allowing lengthening) that is contributed to and then maintained by physical therapy. Thus, it is really the therapy which produces the long-term gains. Some physiotherapists believe that the abnormal motor programmes arising in the UMN syndrome can be inhibited and normal ones facilitated (see Chapter 7); BTX could help this by preventing such abnormal motor activity.

Injection procedure

The most basic goal in BTX treatment is to acheive adequate weakening of the target muscle. Although largely dose dependent, a number of other factors also determine the degree of weakness obtained, which therefore cannot be predicted precisely. In particular, individual sensitivity to the toxin varies markedly. Some average starting doses that are likely to achieve an acceptable response are given in Table 9.5; these may need to be modified for subsequent injections. It should also be remembered that there are two commercial preparations of BTX type A available — Dysport® and Botox® — that have substantially different clinical potencies and thus require different doses; from Table 9.5 it can be seen that the potency ratio between the two preparations is roughly 3–4:1. Our maximum dose is Dysport® 2000 MU and Botox® 500 MU.

THE DOSAGE UNITS BETWEEN DYSPORT® AND BOTOX® ARE THUS NOT INTERCHANGEABLE AND FAILURE TO RECOGNISE THIS COULD POTENTIALLY LEAD TO SEVERE TOXICITY.

EMG also allows accurate placement of the toxin. Intuitively, this seems advantageous although some would argue that large muscles are easily accessible. In our practice, however, we are continually injecting deeper muscles (e.g. tibialis posterior, flexor hallucis longus) and individual finger flexors which demand EMG guidance.

Table 9.5 Common doses of botulinum toxin

Muscle	Dysport® (MU)	Botox® (MU)
Upper limb		
Biceps	300–500	100–150
Triceps	150–250	50–80
Brachialis	100–200	30–75
Brachioradialis	100–200	30–75
Flexor carpi radialis/ulnaris	80–200	30–75
Flexor digitorum superficialis/profundus	80–250*‡	30–100
Intrinsic hand muscles	40–100	10–30
Flexor pollicis longus	30–80	10–25
Lower limb		
Quadriceps	1000–1500*	400–500*
Thigh adductors	1000–1500*	400–500*
Hamstrings	1000–1500*	400–500*
Tibialis posterior	300–500	100–150
Gastrocnemius (medial, lateral)	200–500†	75–150†
Soleus	200–500	75–150
Flexor hallucis longus	100–200	30–75
Flexor digitorum longus	100–200	30–75
Flexor digitorum brevis	200–300	75–100
Tibialis anterior	100–250	30–75
Extensor hallucis longus	100–150	30–50

* Total divided into several sites; † per muscle belly; ‡ individual fascicles may require much less.

There are a number of issues regarding the injection technique, including optimal dilution of toxin, site of injection (search for end-plates?) and number of injection sites per muscle. The need for EMG to guide the injection is also controversial. Assuming no diagnostic information is required, EMG is probably unnecessary for accurate injection of large, readily accessible muscles. This question has not been put to trial in limb muscles. Some injectors believe that the use of EMG (in cervical dystonia) allows a substantially lower dose of BTX. We routinely use EMG, even when muscles are large and accessible, mainly because of the diagnostic information obtained.

Injections are given through a 23 G needle that allows simultaneous recording and injection (Myoject, TECA). We use a dilution (with normal saline) of Dysport® 200 MU/ml (2.5 ml) and Botox® 50 MU/ml (2 ml). No attempt is made to search for end-plates, but injections are usually given in the end-plate region of the muscle, according to anatomical studies. For many muscles, this is in the mid-belly. Small muscles usually receive single-site injections whereas larger muscles (e.g. hamstrings, thigh adductors) receive between two and six. Long muscles such as tibialis anterior, flexor digitorum longus and flexor carpi ulnaris may be prone to a 'compartmentalisation' effect. Poor diffusion away from the injection site produces a marked local denervation. EMG at this site during a maximal voluntary contraction at a follow-up injection often shows a very poor interference pattern, despite quite good strength. This can be avoided by injecting at several sites along the length of the muscle and choosing different sites each time, rather than at the anatomical landmarks recommended by books. The approach to the muscle may need to be such that it minimises unwanted spread of the toxin. For example, a medial approach to brachioradialis is preferred over a lateral approach in order to reduce risk of weakening the adjacent extensor carpi radialis and a resulting wrist drop.

Anatomical guides are helpful for the initial placement of the needle (see charts in Appendix). Confirming that the needle is in the correct place can be done in several ways. The first two require EMG and involve voluntary contraction of the muscle or passive stretch of the muscle looking for a stretch reflex. In each case a sharp, crisp EMG signal is sought. The third is through passive movement of the muscle, observing for needle movement, and the fourth involves electrically stimulating the muscle through the needle and looking for the relevant movement. Patients with the UMN syndrome may not have voluntary control of the muscles and a stretch reflex may not be elicitable. The fourth technique I have found less useful because the stimulation tends to either be poorly localised, so that other muscles are also directly stimulated, or else the main nerve trunk is stimulated with the same result. For some sites (e.g. sole or palm), the injection is so painful that we sometimes will not try to find the best EMG signal and inject as near as possible to the muscle, trusting that diffusion of the toxin will be adequate.

The side-effects are listed in Table 9.6. In practice very few side-effects, other than temporary weakness, are seen. This occurs more

Table 9.6   Side-effects of botulinum toxin

- Excessive weakness with reduced function
- Unintentional weakness of adjacent muscles
- Local pain or haematoma
- Flu-like illness
- Neuralgic amyotrophy-like illness
- Long term – secondary clinical resistance

often in the upper limb and is uncommon in the lower limb. One caution is against vigorous stretching after injection as we have seen a case of intramuscular tear and haematoma in the calf. As with dystonia, there is always the potential risk of secondary non-responsiveness (clinical and biological resistance), through immune or other mechanisms.[10] Those muscles at risk would be those repeatedly given large doses (e.g. hamstrings, thigh adductors). So far we have not encountered this problem.

Post-injection physiotherapy and follow-up

We believe that active physiotherapy after injections of BTX is beneficial. This remains to be proven by a controlled trial but makes good sense. Techniques include stretching exercises, splinting or casting to maintain muscle length and use of an ankle–foot orthosis (AFO). The need for splinting or casting is usually assessed 2 weeks or so after the injection to allow time for the maximum biological (weakening) effect to occur. Sometimes, splinting has not proven necessary; in one case following finger flexor injection, the response was so good with additional release of finger extensor function that it allowed active finger flexor lengthening. We routinely see all patients 3 months after injection to review the response and to determine whether another injection is required. If the initial injection fails to produce sufficient muscle weakness, we prefer not to give a 'booster' injection, because of the risk of antibody-mediated resistance. Rather, we would wait until 3 months after the first injection and repeat with a higher dose. The doses given at subsequent sessions will depend in part on the response to the previous injection and the apparent need at the time. The need for and timing of subsequent injections is difficult. A clear reversal of the gained benefit would be an indication but where improvement is continuing, we tend not to re-inject. We also tend not to re-inject when the original goal has been achieved; these patients are kept under review with continuing physiotherapy until the benefit regresses or it seems apparent that further injections would be beneficial.

CASE HISTORIES

The following case histories illustrate some of the principles of goal setting, BTX treatment and outcome measures, discussed in earlier chapters.

Case 1

A 22-year-old man (AH) made a good recovery after an incomplete traumatic spinal cord injury at the level of C5/6, except for his right hand.[11] He reported difficulty in tasks requiring opening of the hand, for example handshaking, grasping door handles and large objects, and holding the banisters to steady himself when coming down stairs. Examination revealed increased tone in the finger and thumb flexors with minimal extension when the wrist was extended (Fig. 9.3). EMG recordings confirmed the spasticity in the finger and thumb flexors with some voluntary activity of the finger extensors.

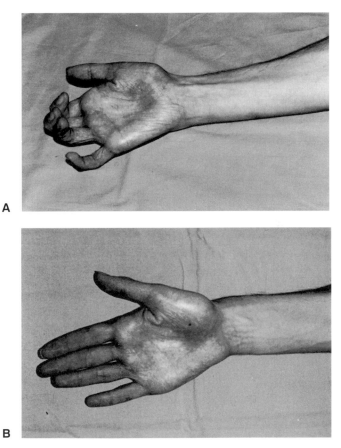

A

B

Fig. 9.3   *Case 1.* **A**. The finger flexors are hypertonic with limited active finger extension; hand function was poor. **B**. Following botulinum toxin, tone was much reduced and active range increased, with improved hand function.

The clinical problem was reduced hand function due to overactivity of finger and thumb flexors. The patient's identified treatment goal was to be able to shake hands in a normal fashion and to be able to reach out and grasp a glass. Treatment sub-goals identified by the clinicians were to weaken the finger flexors in order to reduce tone and to strengthen the finger extensors.

The objective measurements focused on hand function and included a measure of grip strength (the Jamar grip meter), a measure of motor impairment in the hand (the Jebsen hand function assessment) and a measure of focal disability (the nine-hole peg test and the Rivermead motor assessment scale for the upper limb). Measurements of ROM (goniometry) and the Ashworth Scale of spasticity were also taken. Success of the patient's treatment goals (above) was scored subjectively on a visual analogue scale. BTX (Dysport®) was injected under EMG guidance into flexor digitorum superficialis (100 MU) adductor pollicis (50 MU), flexor pollicis brevis (40 MU) and opponens pollicis (20 MU). The measurements were taken at 3, 6, 9 and 12 weeks post-injection.

The measurements revealed weakening of the finger flexors with reduction in tone and increased range of active movement (Fig. 9.3) and the patient's functional treatment goals were achieved. These goals and tone reduction were sustained at 12 weeks despite recovery of full strength in the injected muscles.

Case 2

A 38-year-old woman (TH) was seen 5 months after stroke which had produced a left hemiplegia. The presenting complaint was an inability to place the left foot flat on the floor, making walking impossible (Fig. 9.4). The following problems were identified:

1. Loss of passive range of movement at the ankle joint
2. Soft tissue changes and spasticity in the plantar flexors and invertors of the left foot (confirmed by EMG)
3. Inability to place the foot flat on the floor (a positive support reaction)
4. Pain on standing on the lateral border of her foot.

The patient's treatment goal was to be able to walk again. After discussion, this was modified to being able to walk indoors with the aid of a walking stick and an ankle–foot orthosis. Treatment sub-goals included a reduction in tone of the ankle plantarflexors and increased range of passive ankle movement. Outcome measures

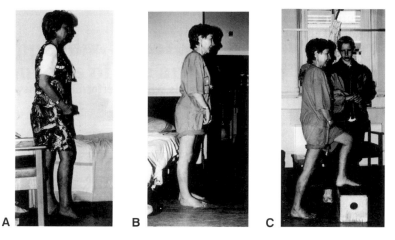

Fig. 9.4 *Case 2.* **A.** A positive support reaction preventing the heel from reaching the ground by several centimetres and interfering with standing and walking. **B.** A reduction in tone in the ankle plantarflexors after botulinum toxin injection with an increased range of movement at the ankle allowing the heel to strike the floor, and even some degree of dorsiflexion by leaning forward (**C**).

included the Ashworth Scale, ROM (goniometry), a timed 10-metre walk and the Rivermead motor assessment scale for the trunk and lower limb. Injections of BTX (Botox®) were given under EMG guidance as follows: medial gastrocnemius (100 MU), lateral gastrocnemius (100 MU), soleus (75 MU), tibialis posterior (100 MU). The patient's goal and the treatment sub-goals were subjectively achieved and supported the outcome measures.

CONCLUSION AND FUTURE DIRECTIONS

BTX appears to be an effective and safe method for the temporary reduction of focal spasticity which has many advantages over the alternatives. However, there is still a large number of unanswered questions. Leaving aside the technical points, which are common to all conditions treated with the toxin, these include the following:

- Can BTX improve function?
- Can BTX produce sustained benefits after a single injection?
- Long-term results of repeated injections?
- Selection of patients, particularly for functional goals?
- Timing of initial and subsequent injections?
- Prediction of reduction in tone (neural versus biomechanical)?

MUSCLES OF THE FOREARM: LATERAL VIEW — DEEPER MUSCLES OF THE FOREARM

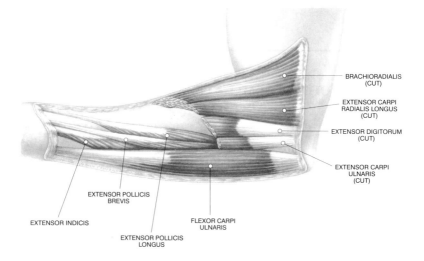

BRACHIORADIALIS
(CUT)

EXTENSOR CARPI
RADIALIS LONGUS
(CUT)

EXTENSOR DIGITORUM
(CUT)

EXTENSOR CARPI
ULNARIS
(CUT)

EXTENSOR POLLICIS
BREVIS

EXTENSOR INDICIS

FLEXOR CARPI
ULNARIS

EXTENSOR POLLICIS
LONGUS

MUSCLES OF THE FOREARM: MEDIAL VIEW — DEEPER MUSCLES OF THE FOREARM

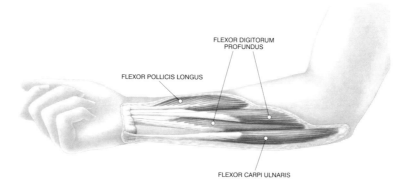

FLEXOR DIGITORUM
PROFUNDUS

FLEXOR POLLICIS LONGUS

FLEXOR CARPI ULNARIS

MUSCLES OF THE ARM: POSTERIOR VIEW — DEEPER MUSCLES OF THE ARM

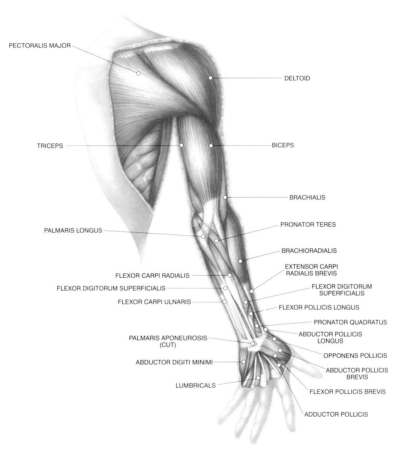

PECTORALIS MAJOR

DELTOID

TRICEPS

BICEPS

BRACHIALIS

PRONATOR TERES

PALMARIS LONGUS

BRACHIORADIALIS

EXTENSOR CARPI RADIALIS BREVIS

FLEXOR CARPI RADIALIS

FLEXOR DIGITORUM SUPERFICIALIS

FLEXOR DIGITORUM SUPERFICIALIS

FLEXOR CARPI ULNARIS

FLEXOR POLLICIS LONGUS

PRONATOR QUADRATUS

PALMARIS APONEUROSIS (CUT)

ABDUCTOR POLLICIS LONGUS

OPPONENS POLLICIS

ABDUCTOR DIGITI MINIMI

ABDUCTOR POLLICIS BREVIS

LUMBRICALS

FLEXOR POLLICIS BREVIS

ADDUCTOR POLLICIS

MUSCLES OF THE LEG AND FOOT

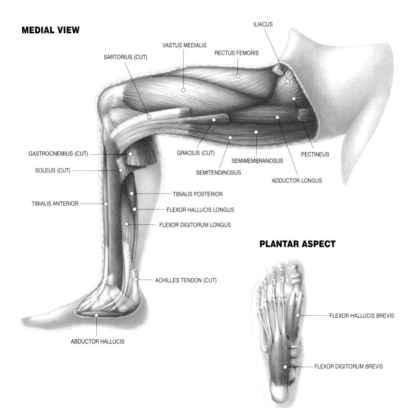

MEDIAL VIEW

ILIACUS

VASTUS MEDIALIS

SARTORIUS (CUT)

RECTUS FEMORIS

GASTROCNEMIUS (CUT)

GRACILIS (CUT)

SOLEUS (CUT)

SEMIMEMBRANOSUS

PECTINEUS

SEMITENDINOSUS

ADDUCTOR LONGUS

TIBIALIS POSTERIOR

TIBIALIS ANTERIOR

FLEXOR HALLUCIS LONGUS

FLEXOR DIGITORUM LONGUS

PLANTAR ASPECT

ACHILLES TENDON (CUT)

FLEXOR HALLUCIS BREVIS

ABDUCTOR HALLUCIS

FLEXOR DIGITORUM BREVIS

MUSCLES OF THE LEG: RIGHT ANTERIOR AND POSTERIOR VIEW

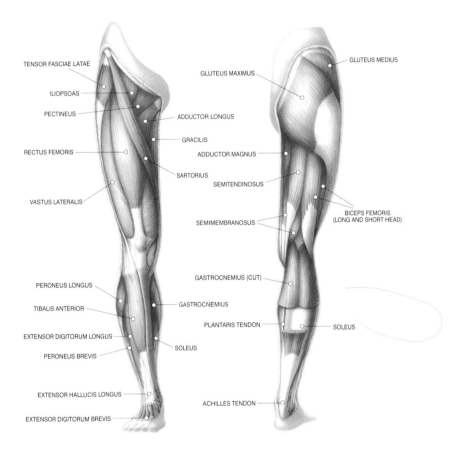

TENSOR FASCIAE LATAE

GLUTEUS MEDIUS

GLUTEUS MAXIMUS

ILIOPSOAS

PECTINEUS

ADDUCTOR LONGUS

GRACILIS

RECTUS FEMORIS

ADDUCTOR MAGNUS

SARTORIUS

SEMITENDINOSUS

VASTUS LATERALIS

BICEPS FEMORIS
(LONG AND SHORT HEAD)

SEMIMEMBRANOSUS

GASTROCNEMIUS (CUT)

PERONEUS LONGUS

TIBALIS ANTERIOR

GASTROCNEMIUS

PLANTARIS TENDON

SOLEUS

EXTENSOR DIGITORUM LONGUS

SOLEUS

PERONEUS BREVIS

EXTENSOR HALLUCIS LONGUS

ACHILLES TENDON

EXTENSOR DIGITORUM BREVIS

Index